D0206595

Migraine

Your Questions Answered

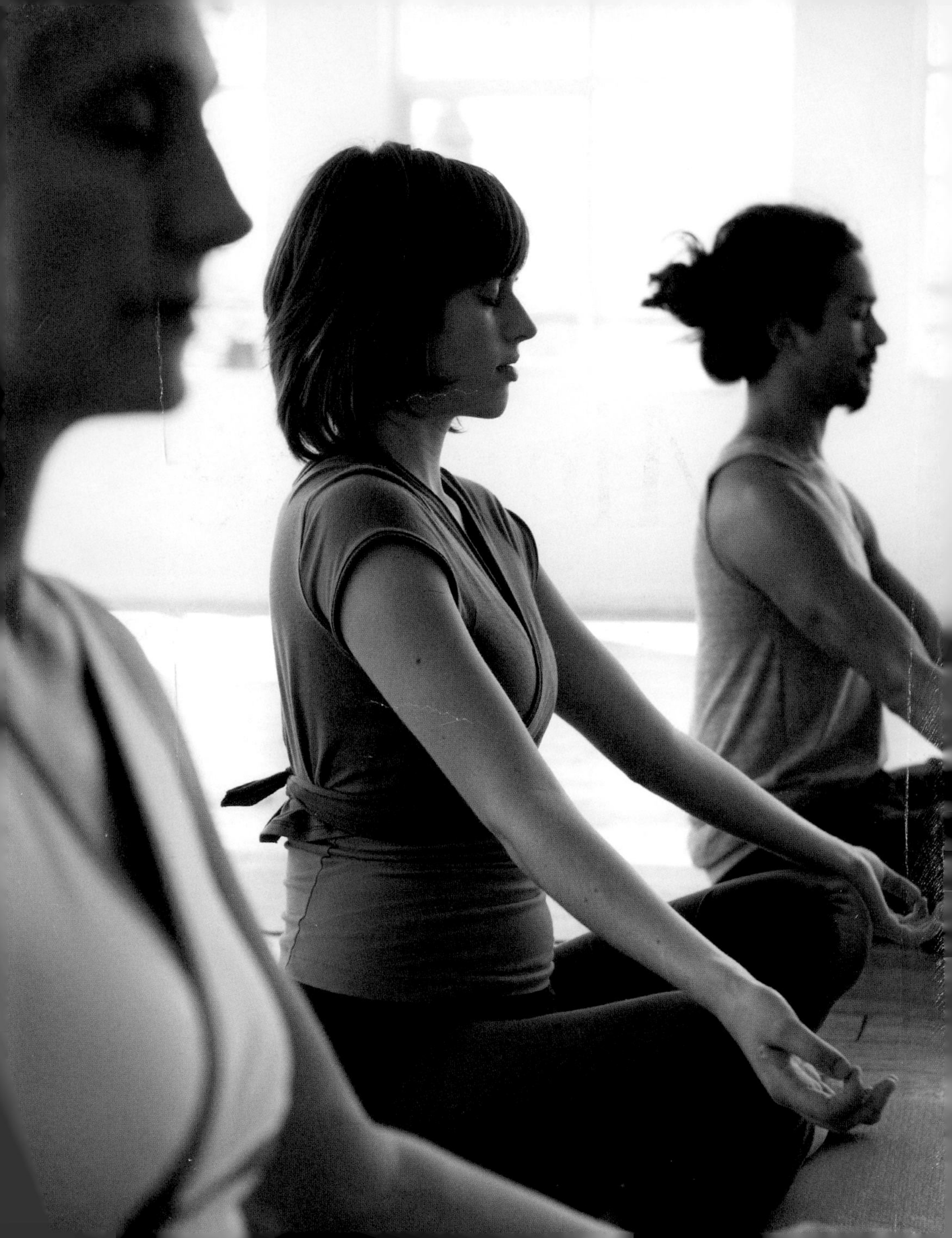

Migraine
Your Questions Answered

Carol A. Foster, MD

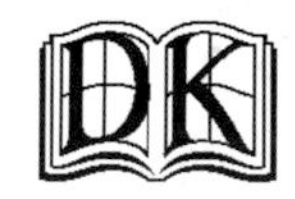

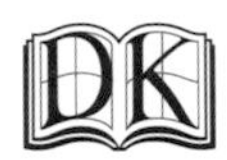

LONDON, NEW YORK, MUNICH, MELBOURNE, DELHI

DORLING KINDERSLEY

Editor Tom Broder
Senior Art Editor Nicola Rodway
US Senior Editor Jill Hamilton
Executive Managing Editor Adèle Hayward
Managing Art Editor Nick Harris
DTP Designer Traci Salter
Production Controller Freya Pugsley
Art Director Peter Luff
Publisher Corinne Roberts

DK INDIA

Senior Editor Dipali Singh
Project Editor Rohan Sinha
Editors Ankush Saikia, Aakriti Singhal
Project Designer Romi Chakraborty
DTP Coordinator Pankaj Sharma
DTP Designer Balwant Singh, Sunil Sharma
Head of Publishing Aparna Sharma

Edited for Dorling Kindersley by
Andrea Bagg and Philip Morgan

First American Edition, 2007

Published in the United States by DK Publishing
375 Hudson Street, New York, New York 10014

07 08 09 10 11 10 9 8 7 6 5 4 3 2 1

MD355—June, 2007

Published in Great Britain by Dorling Kindersley Limited.

A catalog record for this book is available from the Library of Congress.

ISBN: 978-0-7566-2863-5

DK books are available at special discounts when purchased in bulk for sales promotions, premiums, fund-raising, or educational use. For details, contact: DK Publishing Special Markets, 375 Hudson Street, New York, New York 10014 or SpecialSales@dk.com.

Printed in China by Hung Hing

Discover more at www.dk.com

Foreword

Having spent nearly 20 years helping those with migraine to understand their condition and manage attacks, I am well aware of how debilitating the condition can be and how much it can disrupt everyday life. More important, I know what migraine is, not just because I am a headache specialist but because I have migraine too. Ever since my first attack at the age of 12 during a junior high school dance, I have been learning how best to live with migraine and manage my headaches effectively. One thing I can assure you is that there are always steps you can take. It may not always be easy—having a chronic illness never is—but you will come to understand that you can control your headaches.

During my career I have been blessed with the opportunity to be a part of so many special individuals' lives. I hope that in some way I was able to help them understand how truly treatable this condition is. I have written this book in the hope that I can help even more people to use this information in their lives. With the right response and treatment, you can live the life you were meant to live without having headaches stop your dance.

Carol A. Foster, MD

Founder, Valley Neurological Headache and Research Center, Phoenix, AZ

Contents

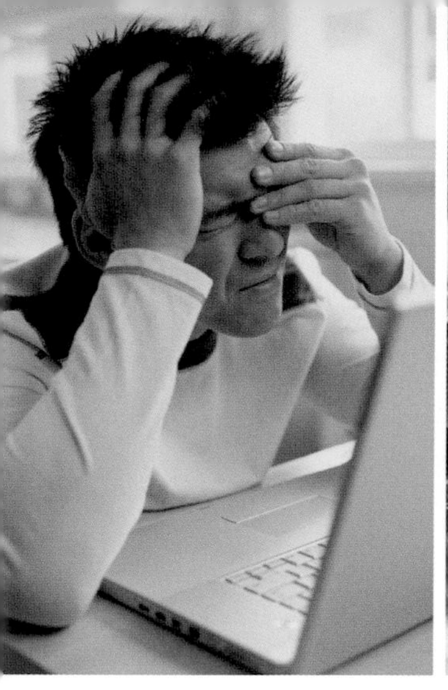
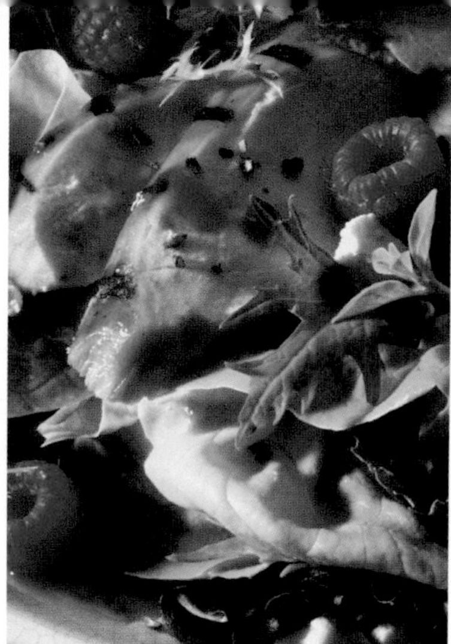
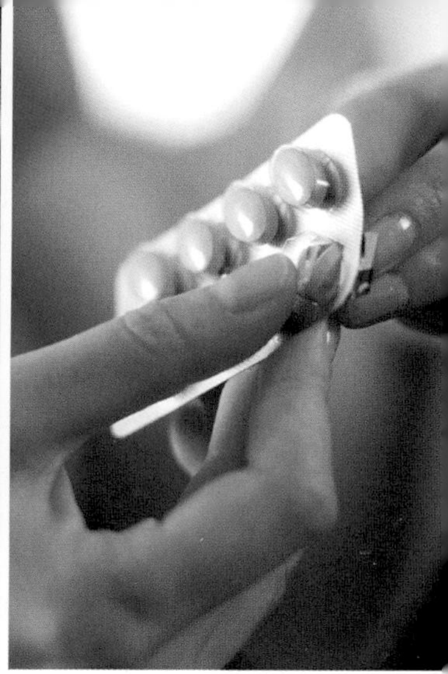

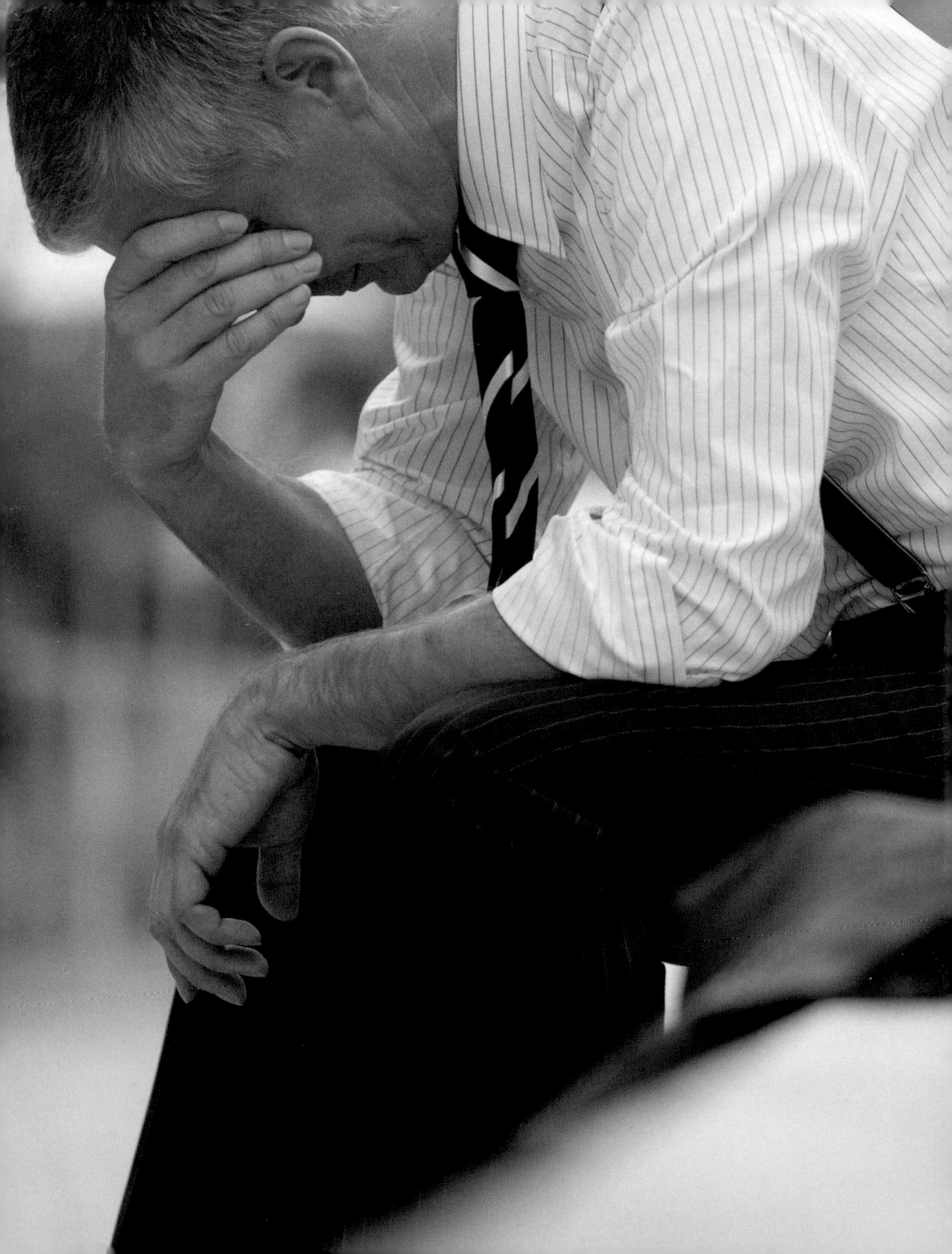

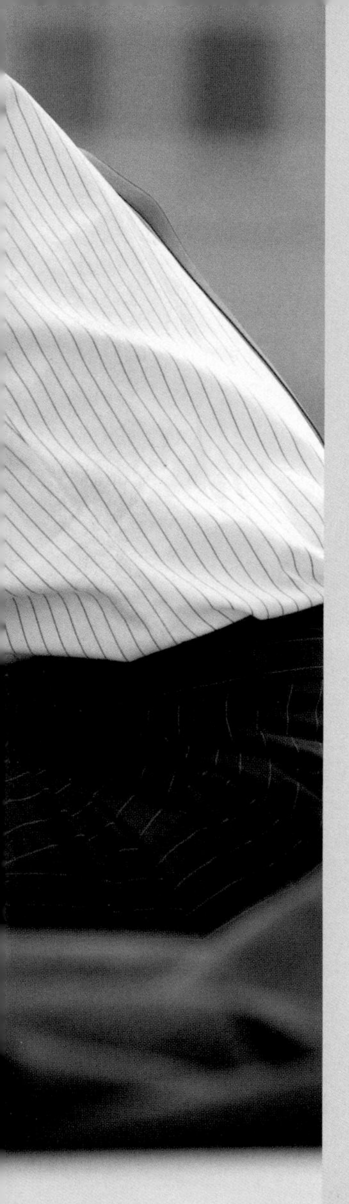

Understanding migraine

People who suffer from intermittent attacks of migraine know the symptoms all too well, the inconvenience of unexpected attacks, the frustration of "cures" that have not worked, and the expense of lost work and healthcare. Understanding migraine—the different types, the symptoms, and the possible causes—gives you the knowledge to deal more effectively with your condition.

What is migraine?

Q I get headaches, so do I need to read a book about migraine?

Having an occasional headache is normal and is unlikely to be a sign that anything is wrong. However, recurrent headaches are not normal and are most commonly caused by migraine. Migraine may not be life-threatening, but it is a chronic (long-term) illness that causes significant suffering and disability for millions of people. This book will help you judge whether your headaches are caused by migraine, and will show you how migraine headaches can be managed.

Q What exactly is migraine?

Migraine is a medical condition that causes intermittent attacks of headache and is associated with nausea and/or vomiting and sensitivity to light, sound, or smells. Like asthma and epilepsy, migraine is considered a chronic medical disorder. Migraine does not always receive as much attention and respect as other medical conditions, because headaches are such a common symptom. But it is important to understand that migraine is a real illness because this will help you accept that your condition deserves the same aggressive treatment as any other chronic disorder.

Q How can something so common be so disabling?

Migraine is much more than a common headache. Migraine is a real, and very treatable, condition that seriously affects millions of individuals worldwide. For years migraine was considered by many to be simply a reaction to stress. Now we have a better understanding of what migraine is, who suffers from migraine, and how to prevent and treat migraine attacks.

Q How do I know if I have migraine or a "regular" headache?

You can tell you have more than a "regular" or tension (stress-related) headache by how disabling the headache is and the symptoms that are experienced with it. In migraine, the headache can interfere with normal activities and there are typical episodes of symptoms that last for a period, then disappear. These symptoms include nausea and/or vomiting and sensitivity to bright light or loud noises. A regular or tension headache is less disabling, although it can still be severe, and is not accompanied by other symptoms. Headaches caused by stress are also more common in those who have migraine (see Tension headache or migraine?, p19).

Q I have bad headaches, but I can live with them. Why should I get treatment?

If your headaches are caused by migraine they are very treatable, and you are missing out on life by putting up with unnecessary pain. Yes, you can often try to ignore the headache or take medications to dull the pain, but what you may not realize is how much your quality of life is affected. More importantly, as you push through the pain, and simply go on living with the headaches, the condition may be getting worse. Eventually, the headaches can affect your whole life, including your job, your social activities, and your relationships.

Q If I have migraine, why can I not simply take a pill for the headaches?

Migraine is a chronic (long-term) illness and cannot be successfully managed unless you have a good understanding of the condition, how it can be treated, and how you may need to change your lifestyle. Managing a chronic illness is never as simple as taking a medication and getting on with life as usual. The idea of having to live with a chronic illness may not be easy, but it is better than living with headaches.

Myth "Migraine is simply a bad headache"

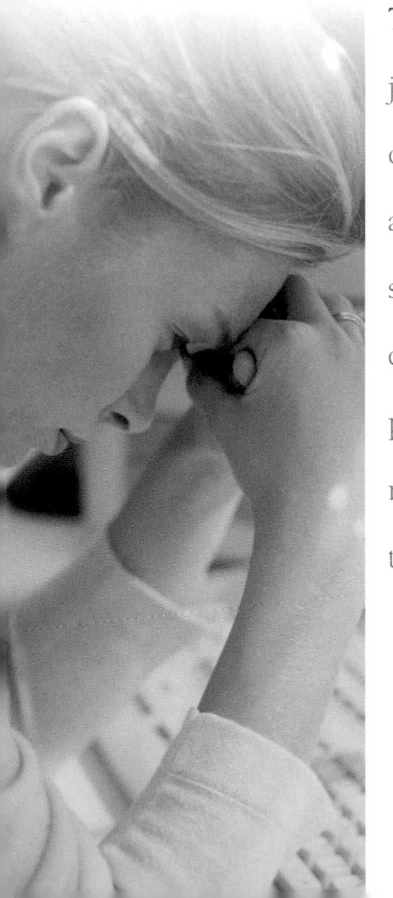

Truth No, there is more to migraine than just a "bad" headache. Migraine is a disorder of the brain, triggered by certain factors, such as stress, and a severe headache is only a symptom of this. Migraine is a progressive condition that is described aptly by the phrase, "a headache begets a headache." The more frequent the migraine attacks become, the more attacks you are likely to have.

Q Why do I have to change my life if the migraine happens only once in a while?

In many ways migraine is similar to asthma and epilepsy. In between attacks of migraine, individuals feel fine. Everyone with a chronic condition must make lifestyle changes treatment to be successful. Chronic disorders like asthma, epilepsy, and migraine are among the most difficult for people to accept in their lives because the symptoms are so intermittent. There is a natural tendency to want to deal with the problem when you experience the attack and ignore the condition when you are symptom-free. The major difficulty with this approach is that you are simply treating the symptoms and not the disease.

Q Will my migraine get worse?

For some individuals with migraine, the attacks can become more severe and more frequent. However, some people have only a few attacks during their entire lifetime. The important point to understand is that you cannot gamble on this fact and ignore migraine if the attacks begin to increase in severity or frequency.

Q Why would the migraine get worse?

Although not all headache experts and neurologists agree, migraine attacks, like epileptic seizures, may become more frequent with each attack, through a process called kindling. Many individuals with migraine go on to develop more frequent headaches. This trend has been termed the transformation of migraine into chronic migraine or chronic daily headache (more than 15 headache days a month). There are many risk factors for the development of chronic daily headache that will be discussed later. Suffice it to say at this point that life is too precious to spend one minute, let alone everyday, suffering from a treatable headache or migraine attack.

The types of migraine

Q What are the types of migraine?

Migraine without aura is the most common type of migraine, accounting for 85–90 percent of all migraines. Only 10–15 percent of individuals with migraine have migraine with aura. There are some migraine syndromes of childhood that may infrequently be experienced by adults. Related headache disorders include tension headache, medication overuse headache, cluster headache, post-traumatic headache, episodic paroxysmal hemicranium, and others (see also pp16–19).

Q Who gets migraine?

Migraine does not appear to target one group of people or another. However, migraine does appear to be inherited: most individuals with migraine can identify a close relative with the condition. Migraine is thought to follow a dominant inheritance pattern (that is, people who inherit the gene for migraine get the condition). Studies show that more women than men report experiencing migraine.

Q Why do more women than men have migraine?

The fact that more women than men experience migraine does not mean that more women have the condition. Studies of children before puberty show that boys are just as likely to have migraine as girls. Perhaps women have more attacks after puberty than men because of the effect of estrogen (the female sex hormone). Population studies use very strict criteria for migraine, and it is likely that many cases of migraine in men and children are missed. Studies of adults with headache have found that the prevalence of moderate to severe headaches not considered as migraine is nearly equal in both genders.

Q How common is migraine?

In any year, nearly 30 million Americans (12 percent of the population) experience migraine. Studies vary little from country to country, with most showing the same prevalence of migraine as in the US. In the American studies, 18 percent of women and 8 percent of men surveyed said they had experienced a migraine attack in the previous 3 months.

Q Can migraine attacks be triggered?

A migraine trigger influences the brain in such a way that it sets off a migraine attack. Just as an asthma attack can be triggered by a cat for someone allergic to cat dander, a migraine attack can be triggered by, for example, a missed meal or a late night. The difference is that a migraine trigger is not caused by an allergy. There are many migraine triggers, both from the external environment and from within the body. Common triggers are stress, lack of sleep, missed meals, menstruation, and foods such as chocolate or cheese. Being aware of your triggers helps you avoid them and control the frequency of migraine attacks.

Q When are people more likely to experience migraine attacks?

Both men and women experience more frequent migraine attacks between the ages of 35 and 45 years. The attacks typically start at a younger age. Boys frequently start having migraine attacks before puberty and get better during and after adolescence. Girls usually start experiencing migraine or have more frequent attacks with the onset of puberty.

Q Can migraine attacks become more frequent at any age?

Yes, men, women, and children can develop more frequent attacks at any age. Migraine is more likely to progress if attacks are not treated. Overuse of medications such as analgesics can lead to chronic daily headache.

Types of migraine

Migraine is the most common type of headache disorder. To help them determine whether someone has migraine and what type it is, doctors use certain criteria set out in the International Classification of Headache Disorders-II (ICHD-II). The following criteria are based on this classification. A diagnosis of migraine is only made when it has been determined that the symptoms are not caused by another illness.

VISUAL DISTURBANCES

The classic visual disturbance experienced during the aura of a migraine attack varies little between individuals. Drawings of migraine visual auras look much the same, even though they may have been drawn more than 100 years apart. It starts with a small area of distorted vision surrounded by bright zigzag lines in the central visual field. This visual disturbance, called a scintillating scotoma, gradually increases in size over time, usually taking 10–60 minutes to fully develop. Although the vision is distorted within the central area, the individual can see clearly around this area. Once the visual disturbance has completely disappeared, the headache and other more typical migraine symptoms usually develop within 60 minutes. Some individuals may experience the visual aura on occasions and not develop a headache.

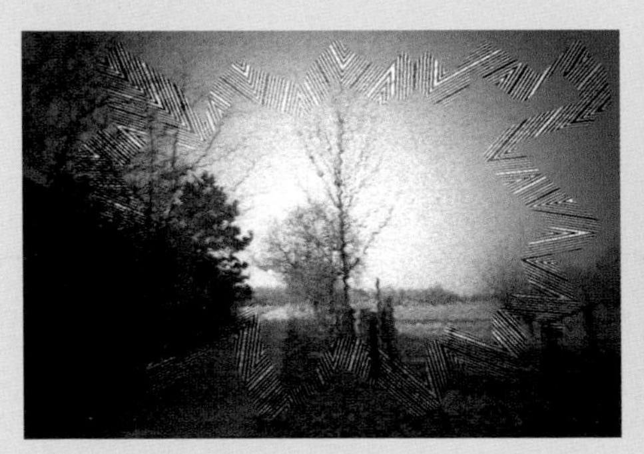

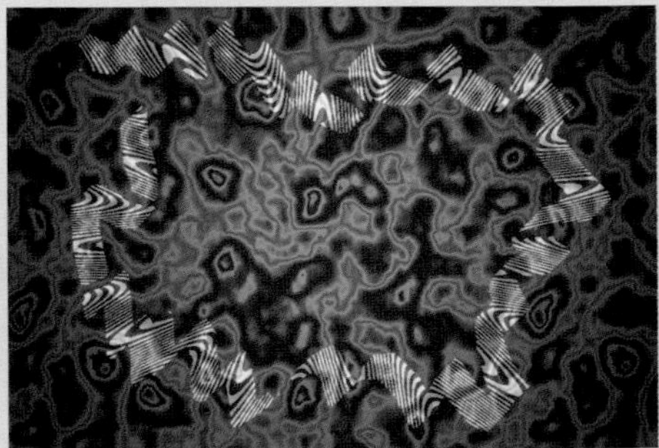

Delia Malchert, Scintillating scotoma, 2002. © 2004 Delia Malchert (http://www.migraene-aura.de/galerie/galerie4.htm, October 25, 2002)

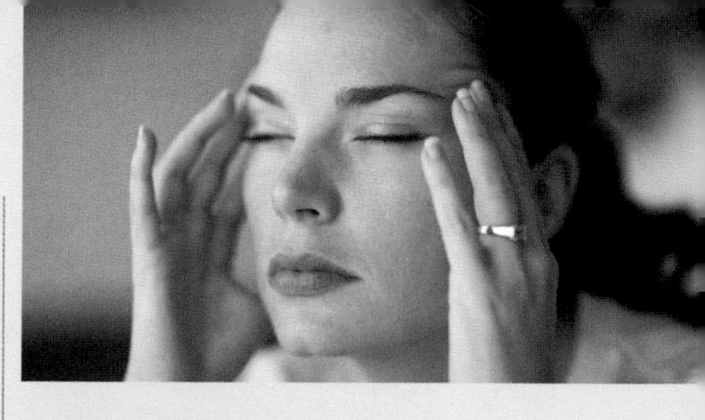

MAIN TYPES OF MIGRAINE

The ICHD-II classification recognizes 2 main types of migraine—migraine without aura and migraine with aura. An aura is a group of symptoms, mainly visual, that develops before the onset of the main headache (see opposite page). Migraine without aura is the most common type of migraine. Only 10–15 percent of people who have migraine experience the symptoms of an aura.

Migraine without aura

① At least 5 attacks, fulfilling ② – ④

② Headache attacks lasting 4–72 hours (untreated or unsuccessfully treated)

③ Headache has at least 2 of the following characteristics:

- One-sided
- Pounding or throbbing
- Moderate to severe intensity
- Aggravation by, or causing avoidance of, routine physical activity

④ During headache at least 1 of the following:

- Nausea and/or vomiting
- Photophobia and phonophobia (conditions in which light and sound are uncomfortable or irritating)

Migraine with aura

① At least 2 attacks fulfilling ② – ④

② Aura consisting of at least 1 of the following but with no paralysis:

- Fully reversible visual symptoms including positive features (seeing flickering lights, spots, or lines) and/or negative features (loss of vision)
- Fully reversible sensory symptoms consisting of pins and needles and/or numbness or loss of sensation
- Fully reversible dysphasic speech disturbance (slurred speech or word-finding problems)

③ At least 2 of the following:

- One-sided visual symptoms and/or one-sided sensory symptoms
- At least 1 aura symptom develops gradually over 5 minutes or more and/or different aura symptoms occur in succession over 5 minutes or more
- Each symptom lasts 5–60 minutes

④ Headache fulfilling the criteria for migraine without aura begins during the aura or follows aura within 60 minutes

MIGRAINE ASSOCIATED WITH MENSTRUATION

Many women have migraine attacks around the time of menstruation. These attacks are often particularly severe and last longer than other types of migraine.

Pure menstrual migraine

① Attacks, in a menstruating woman, fulfilling criteria for migraine with aura

② Attacks occur exclusively on day 1±2 (i.e. days -2 to +3) of menstruation in at least 2 out of 3 menstrual cycles and at no other times of the cycle

Menstrually related migraine without aura

① Attacks, in a menstruating woman, fulfilling criteria for migraine without aura

② Attacks occur exclusively on day 1±2 (i.e. days -2 to +3) of menstruation in at least 2 out of 3 menstrual cycles. They may also occur at other times of the cycle

UNCOMMON FORMS OF MIGRAINE

Migraine attacks associated with atypical neurological symptoms occur infrequently. A complete neurological evaluation is needed to make a diagnosis of basilar artery and hemiplegic migraine.

Basilar artery migraine

① Fulfills criteria for migraine with aura

② Includes 2 or more aura symptoms of the following types:
- Disturbed visual perception, sometimes with visual hallucinations
- Vertigo (dizziness)
- Tinnitus
- Decreased hearing
- Double vision
- Unsteadiness
- Decreased level of consciousness

Hemiplegic migraine

① Fulfills criteria for migraine with aura

② Hemiplegia (weakness or paralysis of the limbs on one side of the body)

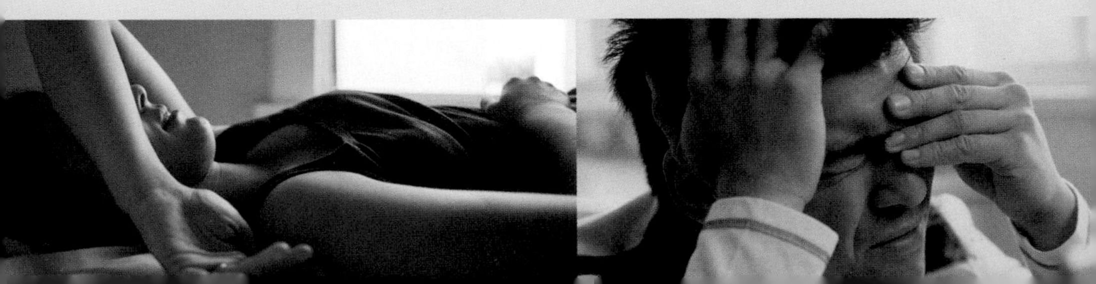

CHILDHOOD PERIODIC SYNDROMES

Several conditions affect children, and a consultation with a doctor is needed to confirm a diagnosis. These conditions are common precursors to migraine in adults.

Cyclical vomiting

① Intermittent episodes of vomiting with intense nausea

② Symptom-free between attacks

Abdominal migraine

① Pain centered around the umbilicus (belly button) with multiple attacks in a day or a few attacks in a month

② Pain may or may not be associated with nausea and vomiting

Benign paroxysmal vertigo of childhood

① Episodes of vertigo (dizziness)

② Between episodes, usually typical migraine attacks consisting of headache

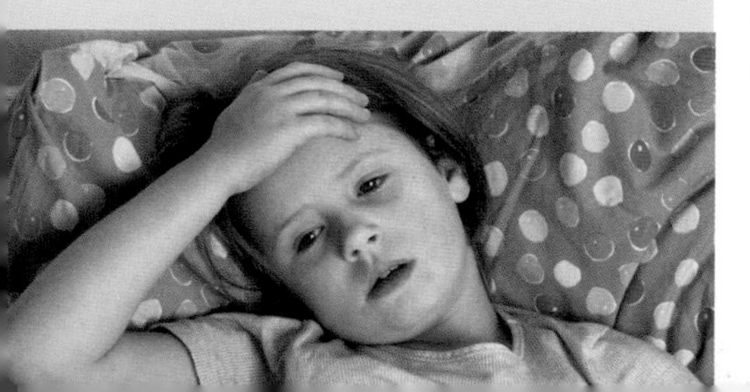

TENSION HEADACHE OR MIGRAINE?

When making a diagnosis of migraine, doctors will use the ICHD-II classification to help them distinguish between a tension-type headache and a migraine headache. A tension-type headache often feels like a band of pressure but does not have the same associated symptoms as migraine.

The following sets out the criteria for a tension-type headache:

- At least 10 headache episodes occurring on less than 1 day per month on average, and fewer than 12 days per year.
- Headache lasting from 30 minutes up to 7 days.
- Headache that demonstrates at least 2 of the following features: it affects both sides of the head; it has a pressing or tightening (but nonpulsating) quality; it is of mild to moderate intensity; it is not aggravated by routine physical activity.
- No nausea or vomiting.
- Associated with either photophobia or phonophobia (in which light or sound are uncomfortable or irritating) but never both.

Causes and symptoms

Q What causes migraine?

Migraine is an inherited disorder of brain chemistry that causes attacks characterized by a complex of symptoms that occur over a period of hours to days. The symptoms of a migraine are caused by a disturbance in brain function related to the brain chemical serotonin. There are many theories to explain the disturbance in brain function but none of them has been proven to date.

Q What is serotonin?

Serotonin is a brain chemical known as a neurotransmitter. Neurotransmitters control brain activity by regulating the electrical activity of brain cells (neurons). Serotonin and other brain chemicals function like traffic lights, allowing electrical impulses to jump from one brain cell to the next at the right time. Serotonin acts like a red light, and another brain chemical, epinephrine, acts like a green light. Together, these brain chemicals modulate or control brain cell activity.

Q How does a problem with serotonin relate to migraine?

Serotonin plays a key role in controlling brain cell activity, and it is believed that disturbances of brain function associated with the start of a migraine attack may be related to an abnormality in the functioning of serotonin. However, researchers disagree about which part of the brain is involved in the process of a migraine attack and how serotonin is involved. What we do know is that the most effective medications used to stop a migraine attack are serotonin medications, which affect the serotonin receptors (structures on the cell surface to which serotonin attaches).

Q I've read that migraine is the result of changes in blood vessels. Is this true?

It has been thought that migraine is caused by changes in the size of blood vessels in the brain. Constriction of blood vessels, restricting blood flow to the brain, was thought to cause the symptoms, or aura, that sometimes precedes a migraine attack. After the aura, the blood vessels dilate (enlarge), causing the headache to subside. We now understand that the process is much more complicated.

Q What is the current theory for the cause of migraine?

One current theory proposes that serotonin-controlled nerves from the brain stem activate receptors, or "switches," on blood vessels. The brain stem connects the brain to the spinal cord. In addition to all the nerves that run throughout the spinal cord, it contains the pain control system, the sleep control system, the balancing system, and the vomiting center. Activation of nerves in the brain stem causes the blood vessels to leak fluid and chemicals, causing the headache. This theory is called the brain stem generator (BSG) theory for migraine.

Q Does the BSG theory explain everything about migraine?

The problem with the BSG theory is that it doesn't explain the other symptoms of migraine apart from headache, or why certain environmental changes trigger a migraine. Another theory is that migraine results from an abnormality in how brain cells function in the brain stem, hypothalamus (a part of the brain that controls automatic body processes), and other areas of the brain. This theory is based on the observation that in those with migraine, brain cells appear to be hyperexcitable (overly responsive to stimulation). It is not yet known whether this hyperexcitability is caused by a problem with serotonin or whether it is a problem related to genetic differences in the brain cells themselves.

Q Could the cause of migraine be explained by all of the theories combined?

Yes, it is possible that abnormal serotonin levels could cause hyperexcitability of brain cells that in turn triggers the brain stem to cause the headache of a migraine attack. As technology gives us improved ways to research brain cell chemistry, we can understand better how a migraine attack occurs and how the condition is inherited. The most important consequence of research is the development of new treatment options.

Q How does abnormal brain activity cause the symptoms of a migraine attack?

Disruption of brain cell activity causes a wave of electrical activity that moves across the brain, causing all of the symptoms of a migraine attack. Think of it as a disruption in the electrical grid system of a major city. A domino effect causes one system to "short-circuit" the next system.

Q How does understanding what causes my migraine help me with my treatment program?

When you know what causes migraine, you have a better understanding of how your treatment program helps you control the migraine attacks. If you know that abnormal serotonin and hyperexcitable brain cells are likely factors in migraine, you will understand why your doctor suggests certain treatments or lifestyle changes. For example, you may be given medication that affects serotonin activity or be asked to do relaxation exercises to help reduce hyperexcitability of brain cells.

Q How do I deal with people who do not understand my condition?

People with migraine sometimes find that family, friends, or coworkers do not understand the condition and may think they are just making a fuss about "regular" headaches. If you are familiar with the causes of migraine, you can share this information and help others more fully understand your illness.

Q Does everyone with migraine get the same symptoms?

A range of symptoms occurs during a migraine attack, and appear in a particular sequence (see box below). However, not everyone experiences all of the symptoms, and individuals may experience different symptoms with each migraine attack.

SEQUENCE OF SYMPTOMS IN A MIGRAINE ATTACK

Understanding that a migraine attack is actually a sequence is important because it makes you realize that migraine is not simply a bad headache. The sequence of migraine symptoms has been described as having 3–4 distinct but overlapping phases: the prodrome, the aura (when present), the headache, and the postdrome. Each phase has particular symptoms that may overlap and continue into the next phase. Understanding the symptoms of a migraine attack helps you take action early enough in the attack to successfully treat and stop the process.

THE PHASES OF A MIGRAINE ATTACK

The Prodrome Phase (duration 12–24 hours)

- Increased appetite • Decreased appetite
- Food cravings • Constipation • Fatigue
- Irritability • Swelling of hands and feet
- Increased yawning • Depressed mood
- Difficulty concentrating

The Aura Phase, when present (duration 10–60 minutes)

- Visual disturbances • Numbness
- Difficulty speaking • Vertigo
- Clumsiness • Mild paralysis

The Headache Phase (duration 2–72 hours)

- Headache • Nausea and/or vomiting
- Light and/or sound sensitivity
- Sensitivity to smells

The Postdrome Phase (duration 12–24 hours)

- Elevated mood (euphoria)
- Depressed mood • Irritability
- Fatigue • Diarrhea
- Increased urination
- Food intolerances

Q What are the warning signs that an attack has started?

The warning signs that a migraine headache may develop are the symptoms of the first and second phases of a migraine attack. The symptoms may vary from individual to individual and may or may not occur before the headache. People may also experience the symptoms of the initial phases without progressing to the headache. One theory suggests that the symptoms of a migraine attack are caused by a wave of electrical disturbances in the brain, and therefore the symptoms may not appear if the wave is interrupted.

Q What symptoms might I experience during the initial, or prodrome, phase?

During the initial, or prodrome, phase of a migraine attack you may experience changes in appetite, either decreased or increased, along with certain food cravings. Your hands and feet may swell, and constipation may be a problem. Mood changes, with feelings of anxiety or depression, are frequently present during this phase. Irritability is a prominent symptom that is well recognized by people with migraine and those around them. Fatigue is also common, and you might find yourself yawning excessively. Mental concentration is disturbed, and there is difficulty in spelling or doing simple math or word-finding problems. The duration of the prodrome phase is typically 12–24 hours.

Q What is a migraine aura?

A migraine aura is a group of symptoms that may occur before the onset of a migraine headache. The aura is the second phase of a migraine attack. Only 10–15 percent of people with migraine experience an aura, and in this group, an aura may not occur with every migraine attack. The aura usually lasts for 10–60 minutes and precedes the headache by 20–30 minutes.

Q What is the most common symptom of the aura phase?

The most common symptom is a visual disturbance called a scintillating scotoma (see p16). It manifests itself as a curved area of visual disturbance surrounded by bright zigzag lines called fortifications. There may be either total loss of vision or simply visual distortion. It typically affects central vision and spreads to one side of the visual field. The visual distortion may appear as if one is looking through broken glass or a kaleidoscope. The area of visual distortion increases in size over 10–60 minutes, then disappears, to be followed by the headache phase. Some may develop other temporary neurological symptoms following the visual symptoms and before the headache.

Q Might I experience different symptoms during the aura phase?

Yes, you may experience a range of symptoms during a migraine aura. Visual disturbances include seeing momentary spots of color, black spots, or bright flashes of light. Infrequently, objects may appear to move or change shape or size. Instead of visual disturbances, some people experience a tingling sensation in the arms or around the mouth. Others have difficulty speaking, vertigo, or loss of balance. Some auras include all the mentioned symptoms, with the individual first experiencing visual changes, then speech disruption, and finally sensory symptoms.

Q What is the connection between migraine with aura and patent foramen ovale?

The foramen ovale is a small opening in the heart of a fetus that diverts blood from the right atrium to the left. It usually closes soon after birth but remains open (patent) in some people. Mostly, if this congenital heart defect is minor with no symptoms, then it is left untreated. However, recent studies suggest that people with patent foramen ovale who have migraine with aura may have fewer attacks of migraine after the defect is corrected.

Q What happens in the headache phase of a migraine attack?

The third phase of a migraine attack is the headache phase. The headache is frequently, but not always, one-sided. The headache may occur on both sides of the head, or at the front or the back of the head. More important than the location of the pain is the fact that the pain continues to be fairly typical from one attack to the next. The headache is usually made worse by activity and may be associated with nausea with or without vomiting, and sensitivity to light and sound. The symptoms associated with the headache may vary in severity between different migraine attacks and between different migraine sufferers.

Q What does the headache feel like?

The pain of the headache phase is most often a throbbing pain. However, in some people it can be a steady or squeezing pressure with or without sharp stabbing pains. The headache is made worse by activity, and resting in a quiet, dark room may help to make the person feel better. The headache may last for hours to days. Usually, the headache is of shorter duration in children, often 2 hours or less.

Q What happens in the final phase of a migraine attack?

The final phase is the postdrome phase. Many people describe this phase as a migraine "hangover". It usually lasts between 12 and 24 hours. The most common symptom is mood change, either depression or elevated mood (euphoria). Many people report that they are feeling much better during the postdrome phase because the pain is gone; however, the emotional lift may be a part of the migraine attack. Some people may experience increased need to urinate, diarrhea, and/or food intolerance.

Q What is central sensitization?

Central sensitization is a term that describes how different parts of the brain are involved in the pain process of a migraine attack. As the attack progresses, the pain-control system in the brain stem (which connects the brain to the spinal cord) recruits additional sensory nerves into the pain process. Normally pain is produced only by stimuli that are potentially or actually harmful to the body tissues (noxious stimuli); once these nerves become activated, however, the threshold is lowered. You may experience other painful sensations as well as the headache, often from minor and ordinarily harmless stimuli; these sensations are called cutaneous allodynia (see below) and are a sign that you are developing central sensitization.

CUTANEOUS ALLODYNIA

Cutaneous allodynia (skin hypersensitivity) is defined as pain resulting from a noninjurious stimulus, such as normal heat, cold, or pressure to the skin. The symptoms, which often take the form of extreme irritation or an uncomfortable, painful sensation, typically result from things that are ordinarily innocuous, everyday stimuli. These may include:

- Combing hair
- Pulling hair back into a ponytail
- Shaving
- Rubbing the back of the neck
- Wearing eyeglasses
- Wearing contact lenses
- Wearing jewelry
- Wearing snug or tight clothing
- Using a heavy blanket in bed
- Allowing shower water to hit the face ("it feels like pins and needles")
- Resting the migraine side of the face on the pillow
- Cooking ("the heat is too much")
- Breathing through the nose on cold days ("it burns")

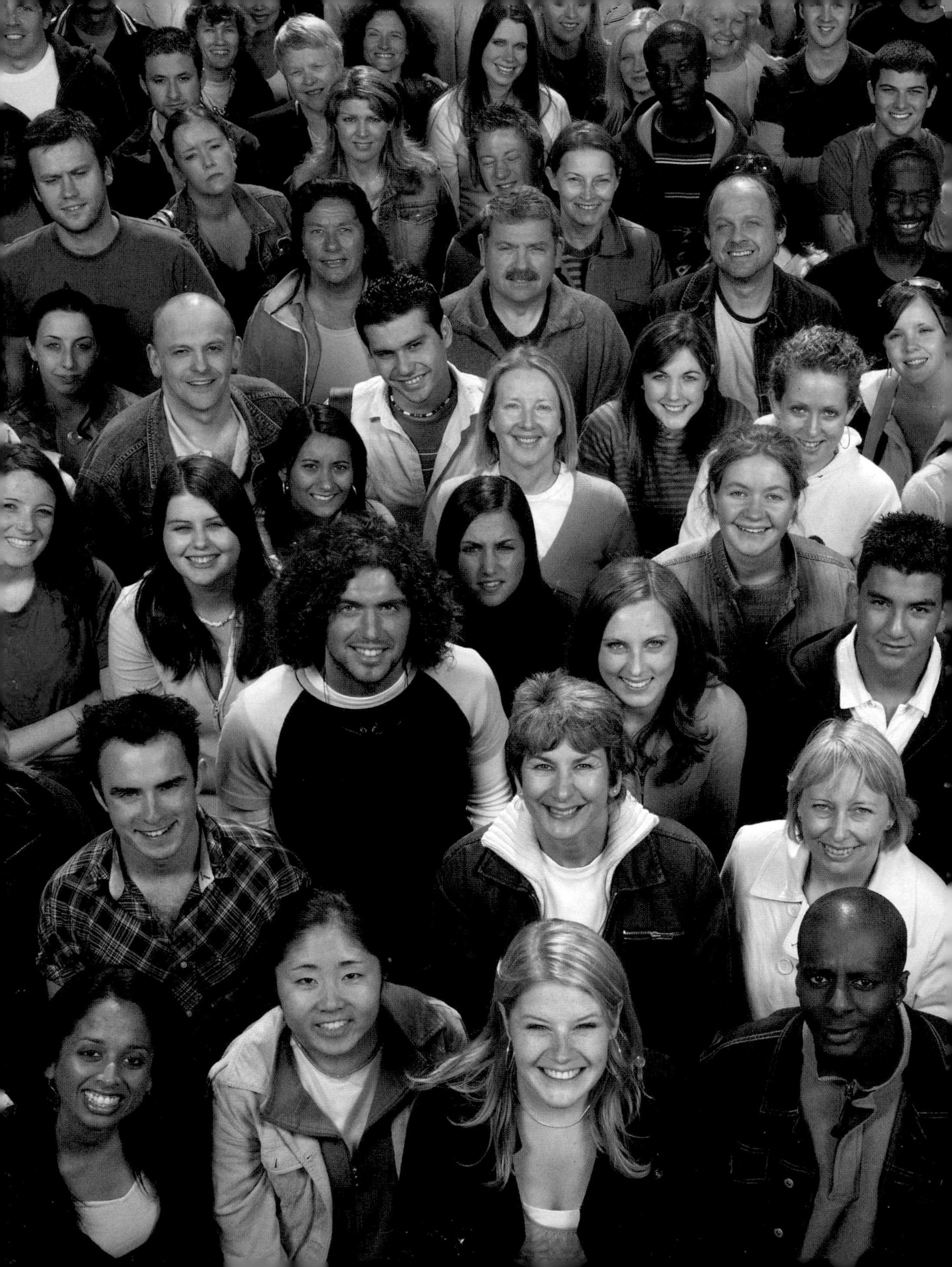

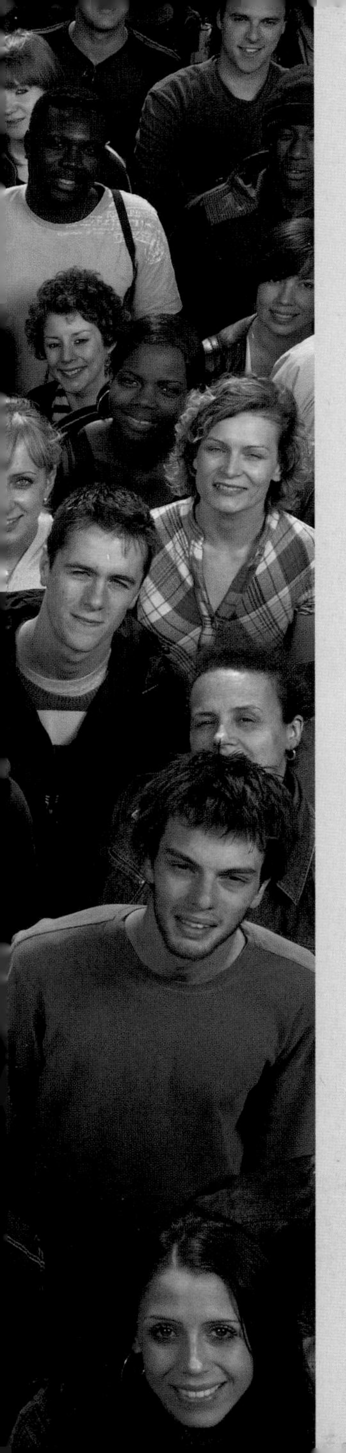

Who gets migraine?

Spanning the great divide of ethnicity, race, nationality, religion, income levels, and gender, migraine is a true equalizer. An inherited disorder, migraine can cause significant disability and lost productivity. It is now ranked by the World Health Organization as number 19 among all diseases worldwide that cause disability. Recognizing how migraine may differ during each stage of life is important for its proper diagnosis and treatment.

Migraine in children

Q Do children get migraine?

Children, both boys and girls, can have migraine. Many adults have their first migraine attack during childhood or during adolescence. However, migraine in childhood is often not recognized and is left untreated until adulthood.

Q Is migraine in childhood different from migraine in adulthood?

Migraine attacks do appear to be different in children. They are usually infrequent and of shorter duration, lasting a couple of hours or less. Children often have abdominal symptoms, known as abdominal migraine, that adults do not experience. When the more typical symptom of headache occurs, it is usually located in the forehead or middle of the head rather than being one-sided. It is rare for children to have the typical aura consisting of visual disturbance that occurs in adults; however, some do describe blurred vision and seeing spots of light or color.

Q What are the symptoms of childhood migraine?

A large percentage, about 70 percent, of children have abdominal pain, sometimes together with nausea and vomiting. This symptom is known as abdominal migraine. When a headache occurs, it is usually located in the frontal area or forehead and is rare in the back of the head. The headache varies in intensity and frequently disappears with sleep. Children may also suffer from bouts of vomiting (cyclical vomiting), episodes of dizziness (benign paroxysmal vertigo), or periods of confusion (basilar artery migraine). Before a diagnosis of migraine is made, the child must be evaluated to exclude other medical problems as a cause for these symptoms.

Q What type of childhood headache could signify a life-threatening problem?

It is rare for a child to awaken with a headache from migraine. The appearance of headache in the morning and headaches in the back of the head must be evaluated by a doctor to rule out other problems, such as a brain tumor. Any headache associated with fever and/or stiff neck must be evaluated to exclude meningitis.

Q What are cyclical vomiting and abdominal migraine?

Children who suffer from cyclical vomiting have periodic episodes of vomiting with intense nausea but are symptom-free between attacks. Abdominal migraine is characterized by pain centered around the umbilicus (belly button), with multiple attacks in a day or a few attacks in a month. The pain may or may not be associated with nausea and vomiting. Children with abdominal migraine usually develop typical migraine during early adulthood.

Q What is benign paroxysmal vertigo of childhood?

Children with this migraine syndrome have episodes of vertigo (dizziness). Between these episodes, they usually have typical migraine attacks consisting of headache. There may be a connection between episodic vertigo and motion sickness because half of all migraine sufferers have experienced motion sickness.

Q What is basilar artery migraine?

The basilar artery supplies blood to parts of the brain involved in vision and balance. In basilar artery migraine, there is a disturbance in this blood flow, resulting in various symptoms. Children with this syndrome experience sudden episodes of confusion and dreamlike states. Some children have an impaired sense of time, a distorted body image, or disturbed visual perception of the environment, with visual hallucinations. The syndrome is sometimes known as the "Alice in Wonderland" syndrome.

Q Do children with migraine need treatment?

Although many adults report experiencing their first migraine attack during childhood or their teenage years, doctors are reluctant to diagnosis migraine in children, particularly since the short-lasting attacks of abdominal pain can be misleading. In addition, they may be concerned that the child may be "labeled for life" as being a migraine sufferer. This view is puzzling, considering that those who care for children do not see a diagnosis of diabetes or asthma in childhood as some kind of label to be avoided. Not making a diagnosis does not make migraine go away. Instead, the child and his or her family are left trying to deal with a problem that has a significant impact on their lives.

Q Why is it so important to correctly diagnose the cause of headache in children?

A headache in a child can indicate a serious underlying problem, such as a brain tumor or epilepsy, so it is particularly important that the child is evaluated promptly by a doctor. If migraine is found to be the cause of the headaches, the child deserves as aggressive a treatment program as an adult. It is not enough to tell the child and parents that "nothing is wrong" or that it is "only migraine" and send them home without treatment. Children with untreated migraine suffer from significant disability; they may have difficulty keeping up with school work and may miss out on social and family activities.

Q Will my child "grow out" of his or her migraine?

Since migraine is an inherited illness, people cannot "grow out" of it. Some children, especially boys, who develop migraine during the first decade of life experience a significant reduction in the frequency of migraine attacks after puberty.

Migraine in adolescents

Q Why do teenagers need to be treated for migraine?

The triggers for a migraine attack are as important for adolescents as for children and adults. Modern society expects a great deal from young people. Their schedules are frequently overcrowded and their diets are often less than ideal. It is very important that migraine is diagnosed and aggressively treated during puberty. Many of the adults treated in headache clinics for chronic daily headache (more than 15 headache days per month) started experiencing symptoms during their teenage years.

Q How do hormonal changes at puberty in girls contribute to migraine attacks?

For most females, the first migraine attack occurs during puberty or a year or two before that. If migraine attacks have started at a younger age, they often increase in frequency the year before menstruation starts. The sex hormones progesterone and estrogen released at puberty not only change the physical appearance of the body but also have effects on brain cell function. It is thought that changes in levels of estrogen are usually responsible for increased migraine in girls around the time of puberty.

Q How do hormonal changes at puberty affect boys with migraine?

For boys at puberty there is a rapid increase in levels of the sex hormone testosterone. For reasons that are not clear, these hormonal changes often lead to a decrease in the frequency of migraine attacks. This does not mean men do not have migraine. Their migraine attacks are more like the attacks seen in children before puberty. Boys appear to have fewer attacks than girls at puberty.

Migraine in women

Q Is migraine more common in women?

Population studies show that prior to puberty, boys have the same number or slightly more attacks than girls. After puberty, girls begin to experience more attacks than boys due to an increase in estrogen levels. Studies demonstrate that more women than men report experiencing migraine. However, since these studies use strict diagnostic criteria for migraine, it is likely that many men with migraine are omitted because their attacks do not always meet these criteria.

Q How can hormones affect migraine?

The hypothalamus in the brain regulates the hormonal changes that occur during a woman's menstrual cycle. The hypothalamus controls the release of hormones from the pituitary gland. Some pituitary hormones in turn control the release of estrogen and progesterone from the ovaries. The coordinated cyclic flow of hypothalamic and pituitary hormones stimulating the release of sex hormones is part of a normal menstrual cycle. A fall in estrogen levels prior to menstruation is believed to lead to migraine attacks.

Q How does menstrual migraine differ from other types of migraine?

Migraine attacks associated with menstruation are particularly severe and last longer than other types of migraine. They usually last 2–3 days, with nausea and vomiting as prominent symptoms. The majority of attacks occur in the 2 days before the first day of menstruation or on the first day of menstruation. The attacks are usually fairly constant, occurring with each menstrual cycle; however, some women may not experience a migraine with every cycle.

Q What about the use of oral contraceptives?

Women who have migraine must avoid the use of oral contraceptives if they have other risk factors for stroke. Migraine without associated risk factors for stroke is not an absolute contraindication for the use of oral contraceptives. The decision to use oral contraceptives must be made in consultation with your doctor.

Q Can I take oral contraceptives to stop menstruation to treat menstrual migraine?

Yes, you can. When you take oral contraceptives without stopping to have menstrual period you prevent the drop in estrogen that triggers a migraine attack. However, you will need to stop taking them intermittently to have a normal cycle. You will also need to discuss this alternative treatment for menstrual migraine with your doctor.

Q Why do so many women in their mid-30s to mid-40s have migraine?

The prevalence or percentage of women in their mid-30s to mid-40s with migraine is much higher than at any other time of life. This is due to hormonal changes, busy lifestyles, and progression of the disease over time. Many women find it a very difficult time to stop and treat their condition because they are so busy. It is important that you do not allow the frequency of the migraine attacks to increase; making time for yourself and the treatment of your illness is therefore crucial.

Q I have tried medications in the past for migraine but I gained weight. Is there a way I can prevent migraine and not gain weight?

Yes, you can. In fact, by following an effective migraine prevention program you are likely to lose weight. Newer medications for migraine prevention are less likely to cause weight gain, and reducing your intake of carbohydrates can reduce headache frequency. Daily exercise helps you control your weight as well as your migraine attack frequency.

Myth "Migraine goes away during pregnancy"

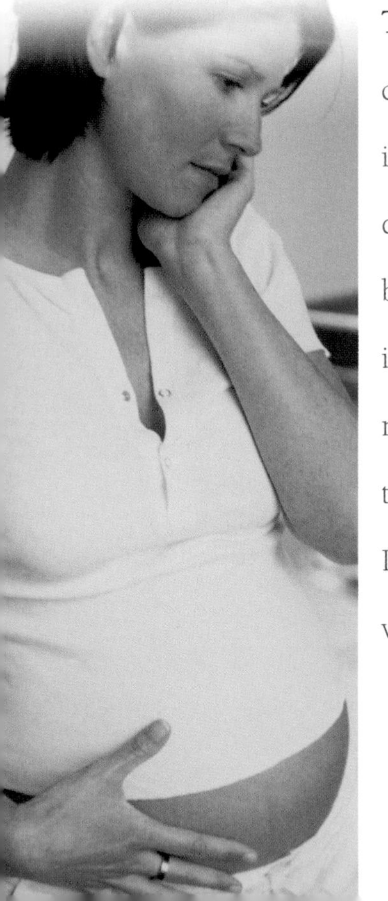

Truth Migraine, especially menstrual migraine, can improve dramatically during pregnancy. It is important to understand, however, that migraine does not just go away. Migraine attacks may become less frequent, but the underlying disorder is always present. Some women actually experience more frequent attacks during pregnancy because they must stop taking medication for the pain. It is very important that your migraine is well controlled before you become pregnant.

Migraine during pregnancy

Q Is migraine different in any way during pregnancy?

It is important to understand that having migraine does not cause harm during pregnancy. Many women with migraine become attack-free during pregnancy. In others, the attacks decrease dramatically, especially during the second and third trimesters. However, not every woman gets better. Some may have more frequent attacks or the frequency of attacks stays the same as before pregnancy.

Q How can I know if my migraine will get better during pregnancy?

Your migraine is more likely to get better during pregnancy if your attacks are associated with menstruation. It is important to control your migraine before pregnancy since most migraine medications cannot be used during pregnancy. Women who often use medications for migraine are likely to have more attacks while pregnant because they must stop their medications.

Q What happens to my migraine after I have the baby?

During the first week following the birth of the baby, approximately 40 percent of women with migraine have an attack. The migraine frequently happens between day 3 and day 6 after delivery. As with menstruation, hormone changes trigger the migraine attack. Sleep disruption, or a change in eating habits or in a woman's schedule related to the baby's arrival, may also act as migraine triggers.

Q Can I take medication for my migraine during pregnancy?

Most medications for migraine must be avoided during pregnancy and breast-feeding. Hence, controlling migraine attacks with lifestyle changes is vital at these times. There are some medications that may be used, but you must consult your obstetrician and pediatrician first.

Migraine in men

Q Why discuss migraine in men, since more women have migraine?

Just because fewer men than women have migraine attacks does not mean that the condition should be ignored in men. Migraine can be controlled if accurately diagnosed and aggressively treated. It is important that both male and female migraine sufferers are educated about their condition and know that help is available.

Q Is migraine different for men?

Yes, migraine may be very different for men, with the symptoms often resembling a sinus or allergy problem. When asked why they waited so long to seek treatment, many male migraine patients say it was because they thought their headaches were due to one of these conditions. In addition, men are also less likely to seek help for any health problem; many men with migraine simply ignore their attacks until they become so frequent that they interfere with work and social life. It continues to amaze me that so many men suffer from recurring disabling headaches without seeking medical help for the problem.

Q Why are men less likely to see a doctor for their migraine?

Men are less likely to go to see a doctor for any condition. Men are more likely to self-diagnose their migraine as a sinus or allergy headache because of associated symptoms of tears forming in their eyes (eye-tearing) or nasal congestion in one nostril. Finally, since migraine still carries with it a certain social stigma, suggesting that individuals with migraine are more "stressed" or less able to handle stress, men may be more reluctant to seek treatment for migraine.

Q Can migraine attacks have different symptoms in men?

Many of the typical symptoms of migraine attacks may be experienced inconsistently or not at all by men with migraine. They often experience a frontal headache and may have associated symptoms of nasal congestion in one nostril and tears forming in one eye (one-sided tearing). Men often experience irritability during their migraine attacks; but nausea, vomiting, or increased sensitivity to light and sound, as often experienced by women, are rare.

Q How often is a sinus headache really a migraine?

One study of nearly 2,400 individuals with "sinus" headache suggested that nearly 88 percent had migraine or probable migraine. In this same study, 28 percent reported experiencing a migraine aura. An aura does not occur with a sinus headache. Many researchers believe that most people, especially men, would rather believe that they have a sinus headache than migraine because of the stigma associated with the latter. It is important that individuals receive an accurate diagnosis from their doctor because many people who incorrectly diagnose themselves with sinus headache end up using medications that may worsen migraine due to medication overuse (see pp78–81).

Q Can I have sinus congestion with a migraine attack?

Yes, you can experience sinus congestion with a migraine. For this reason, migraine is often wrongly diagnosed as a sinus headache. The sinus congestion associated with a migraine is frequently one-sided and is often accompanied by tears forming in one eye (one-sided tearing), a droopy eyelid, and sharp jabs of pain called ice-pick pains. These same symptoms may be found in other primary headache disorders, such as cluster headache and paroxysmal hemicrania.

Migraine and menopause

Q What happens to migraine during menopause?

Menopause and migraine sometimes go well in that migraine attacks decrease in frequency after menopause in most women. However, in some women the frequency of attacks increases in the years preceding menopause.

Q Why does migraine change with menopause?

In the years preceding menopause, migraine attacks can be triggered by changes in estrogen levels just as they are in menstrual migraine. Estrogen plays a significant role in brain cell function, probably as a result of its effect on the brain chemical serotonin. Decreased levels of estrogen at menopause cause symptoms similar to those related to low levels of serotonin. Along with migraine attacks, anxiety and sleep disruption occur.

Q Does migraine get better in a woman after menopause?

Not every woman who has migraine has a decrease in attacks after menopause, especially if the earlier attacks were frequent and not associated with menstruation. Migraine may get worse over time if attacks are not controlled or if certain medications are overused, leading to medication overuse headache (see pp78–81). It is important that migraine be treated with a comprehensive approach instead of waiting for menopause to bring relief.

Q If I have migraine can I use hormone therapy (HT)?

Hormone therapy for menopause is not a simple answer for migraine since estrogen replacement carries with it the risk of other medical problems. Hormone therapy must be discussed with your doctor before starting treatment. Migraine during menopause should be treated in the same way as at any other time during life.

Migraine in elderly people

Q What is migraine like for elderly people?

Both men and women with migraine can expect to see their attacks decrease in frequency in their later years. After menopause, the frequency of migraine attacks significantly decreases unless the individual is experiencing medication overuse headache (see pp78–81) or if migraine was not associated with menopause. If migraine attacks seem to increase or reappear late in life, another medical problem may be aggravating the migraine condition.

Q How can other medical problems in elderly people aggravate migraine?

Medications used to treat medical conditions that commonly occur in elderly people may trigger migraine attacks. Medications for heart disease, high blood pressure, sexual dysfunction, and urinary tract problems are among those that may trigger migraine attacks.

Q Can I start having headaches in my "golden years?"

It is so rare for migraine to start after the age of 55 that the onset of headaches after this age is almost always a signal that another medical condition is present. If you are over 55 and start having headaches it is unlikely, although not impossible, that the cause is migraine. It is very important that you see your doctor about the headaches.

Q If migraine is unlikely then what could cause headaches to start after the age of 55?

Headaches late in life may be associated with life-threatening conditions such as brain tumors, aneurysms (weakened, bulging areas in an artery wall), or inflammation of arteries. General medical problems connected with aging, such as heart disease, lung problems, thyroid disease, and many other illnesses can also be associated with the symptom of headache.

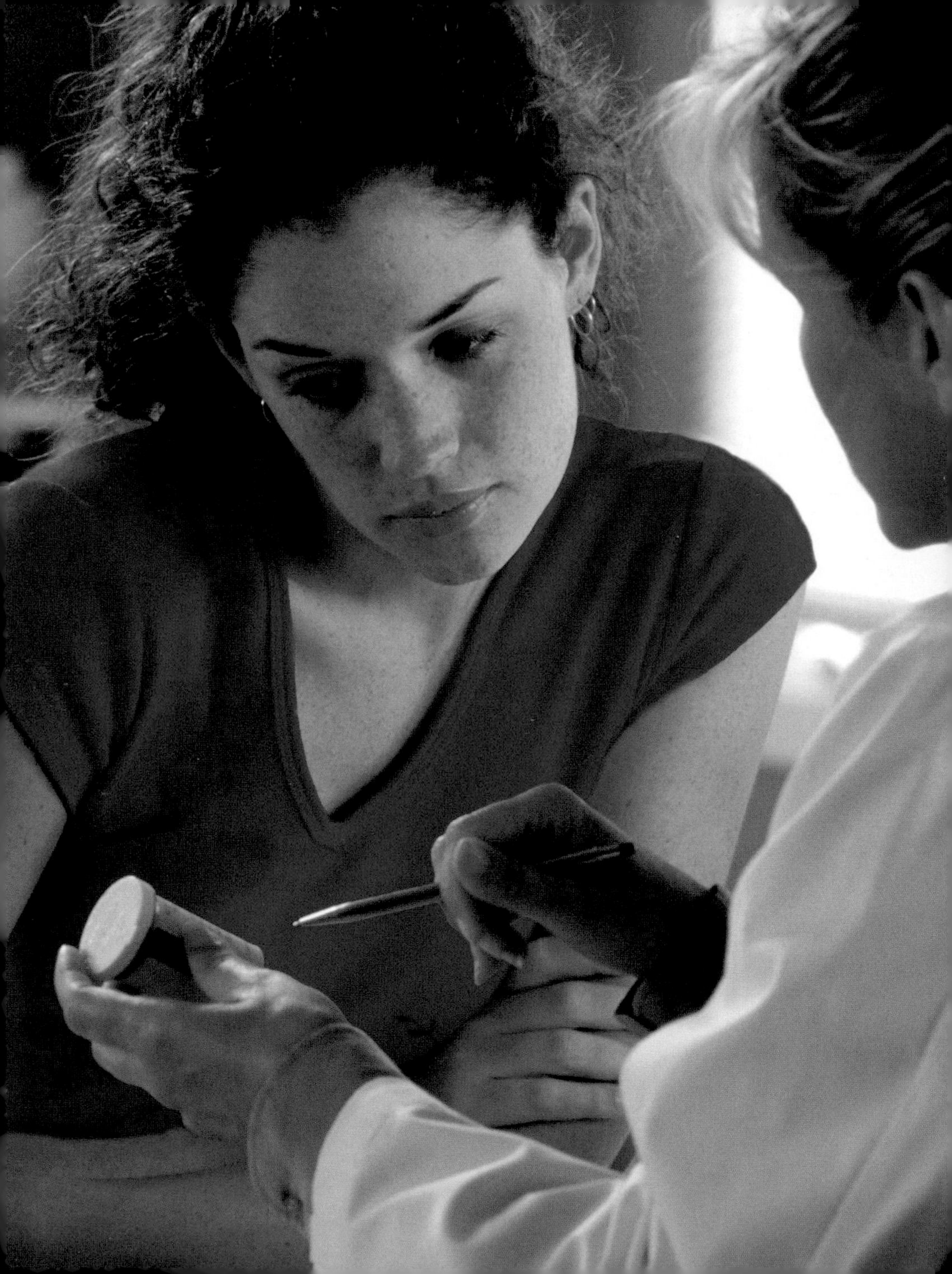

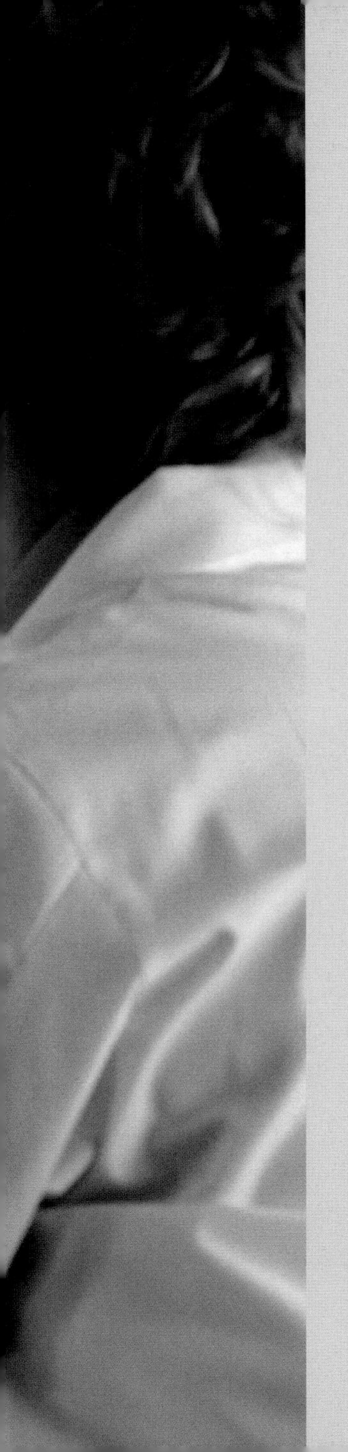

Diagnosing and treating migraine

Migraine can be easily treated, yet less than half of migraine sufferers have been diagnosed or treated. Research has shown that optimal therapy dramatically reduces headache-related disability and prevents the disease from getting worse. Early diagnosis and appropriate treatment are essential.

Diagnosing migraine

Q How is migraine diagnosed?

The diagnosis of migraine is based on your symptoms (see pp16–19), as well as your medical history and that of your family. Recurrent attacks of "sick headaches" lasting 1–3 days in an otherwise well person are most likely to be migraine. If there is any doubt, keep a diary and check with your doctor.

Q Is there a medical test for migraine?

There is no medical test to confirm the diagnosis of migraine. This fact can be frustrating for the individual with migraine. Many people go from doctor to doctor to find out what is wrong with them, and may subject themselves to numerous unnecessary medical tests in the hope of finding something concrete to fix. Fortunately, the typical symptoms and pattern of attacks are usually sufficient to confirm the diganosis. If your doctor does do any tests, it will be to ensure that your symptoms are not the result of an underlying medical problem other than migraine.

Q How do I know if my headaches are caused by migraine rather than another medical problem?

Migraine can cause many symptoms that are related to brain function. It is important that you have a medical evaluation to exclude other disorders as the cause of your symptoms. Rarely, serious conditions such as a brain infection, a brain tumor, or bleeding into the brain can be the cause of headaches and it is particularly important that these are excluded before a diagnosis of migraine is made. Coexisting medical conditions can complicate migraine and must be accurately diagnosed and treated to gain optimal control of migraine (see p45).

Other medical problems

Q How can other medical problems complicate migraine?

Migraine attacks may worsen or increase in frequency if you have another illness. For example, in those with chronic neck and back problems, migraine attacks can be triggered by the pain or by overuse of analgesics and/or muscle relaxants taken for the pain. Apart from being the result of neck pain, migraine may also cause neck pain through a process called central sensitization, in which the nerves become hypersensitive (see p27). Sensitization sets up a terrible cycle of neck pain causing migraine and, in turn, migraine causing neck pain.

Q What do I do if I have neck pain and migraine?

The first thing you need to do is get a correct diagnosis for the neck pain by seeing an appropriate doctor. Once you know what is causing the neck pain, you must avoid any medication for it that would make the migraine worse. It is important to understand that the migraine may be making the neck pain worse, and therefore the migraine must be treated aggressively as well.

Q Can temporomandibular joint problems cause migraine?

No, a temporomandibular joint problem (pain in the head, jaw, and face caused by impaired functioning of the joint where the lower jaw meets the skull) does not cause migraine. Migraine is an inherited problem. However, this problem or any other medical condition can make migraine worse by acting as a trigger for the attacks. Avoiding any medical condition that is a migraine trigger is critical for control of migraine. All pain problems, especially in the neck, face, and head area, must be treated aggressively.

Myth "Most headaches are caused by sinus problems or hormonal changes"

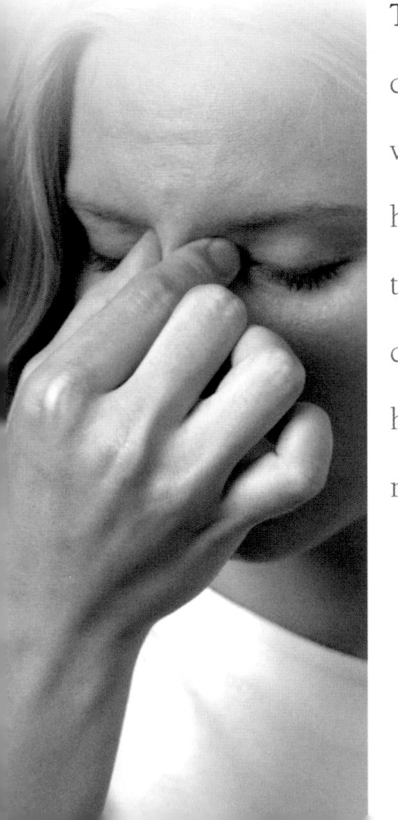

Truth No, migraine is the most common cause of frequent headaches. Most people would rather treat their headaches as "sinus" headaches, and most women will insist that their headaches are caused by hormonal changes. It is a common belief that such headaches are more easily "fixed," and that migraine cannot be treated—which is a fallacy.

Q Could what I think is a neck or temporomandibular joint problem actually be migraine?

Yes, you may be suffering from cutaneous allodynia, in which skin becomes hypersensitive to stimulation (see p27). At the start of a migraine attack, the nerves to the blood vessels in the brain lining are activated, causing the typical throbbing headache. As the migraine attack progresses, the nerves in the brain stem, located at the top of the spinal cord, become activated, producing more discomfort as cutaneous allodynia develops. Neck or face pain may be caused by cutaneous allodynia, which is part of the migraine attack, and missing the diagnosis of migraine would result in the wrong treatment for face or neck pain. Likewise, a misdiagnosis of migraine might miss a neck or temporomandibular problem. An evaluation by an appropriate specialist is required before you start treatment.

Q Can general medical problems cause migraine?

Many medical conditions can worsen migraine and trigger attacks. If you suffer from frequent migraine attacks you must have a general medical evaluation to make sure you don't have other medical problems. Some medical conditions, such as asthma and heart disease, are more likely to trigger migraine attacks than others.

Q What disorders are commonly associated with migraine?

Disorders caused by a problem with the brain chemical serotonin are more likely in someone with migraine. These serotonin-related illnesses include anxiety disorder, depression, bipolar disorder, attention deficit disorder, restless legs syndrome, irritable bowel syndrome, gastroesophageal reflux, insomnia, and fibromyalgia. Other conditions that can trigger migraine attacks include asthma, heart disease, systemic lupus erythematosis, and endocrine problems such as thyroid disease.

Q Can migraine be caused by eyestrain, dental pain, or sinus problems?

Migraine is not caused by eye strain, dental pain, or sinus problems. However, the pain associated with these problems may trigger more frequent migraine attacks. The nerves that go to and from the sinus areas, mouth, and eyes are very complex. These nerves not only contain pain sensory fibers but also nerve fibers that regulate the secretion of fluids such as mucus. When the sensory fibers in a nerve are activated and take information back to the brain, the other fibers in that nerve can also be activated. This complicated process is sorted out in nerve junctions called ganglia in the brain stem. When the sensory nerves send information from eye strain, dental pain, or sinus problems, an overlap of brain cell processing in the brain stem can trigger a migraine attack.

Q How do I know if my symptoms are caused by migraine or another medical problem?

When you have symptoms it is important to go to the appropriate professional to determine the cause of the problem. The place to start is with your own doctor and/or dentist, who will refer you to a specialist if necessary. Pain management for any problem is essential. However, it is important not simply to treat the pain but to address the underlying cause. Using analgesics for a prolonged period of time may cause medication overuse headache if you have migraine, no matter why you are taking the pain pill.

Q What if I have other chronic medical problems in addition to my migraine?

Trying to juggle multiple medical treatment regimens and different doctors is not only confusing but can be expensive. To make sure you get the best response to treatment you must have a doctor who can coordinate your care and healthcare providers.

Preventing migraine

Q Why do I need to prevent migraine attacks?

You must prevent migraine attacks because "a headache begets a headache." Once migraine has been diagnosed, you must start an aggressive treatment program to prevent attacks. Prevention of attacks and stopping attacks quickly is important not just to relieve suffering but also to treat the disease. Without effective treatment, the illness progresses, with attacks becoming more severe and more frequent.

Q How do I get started with my migraine treatment?

The first step is accepting the fact that the condition is part of your life. Treatment for migraine is not dependent upon medication only and requires a change in lifestyle. This is not easy. You must take time to learn about the disorder and be prepared to make the changes required to treat it effectively.

Q How can I make my treatment program successful?

Successful treatment of migraine demands that you make changes to your lifestyle (factors such as diet, exercise, and daily routine) as well as taking medication. Untreated migraine progresses (worsens), causing more disability and interference with work and home life as the years go by. You must make a decision to succeed and persevere with your treatment until you control the migraine attacks. The migraine attacks are an assortment of symptoms that last from a few hours to days. The key to successful treatment is to understand that migraine attacks can be limited in duration and frequency. This can enable you to regain control and get on with your life without fearing the next attack.

Q How can I ask my family, friends, and colleagues to deal with my migraine?

You start by involving them in your treatment. The adjustments required to treat migraine aggressively not only affect the individual with the condition but family, loved ones, and coworkers. Migraine sufferers are often reluctant to make changes, fearing the reaction of others to their condition. However, once those around you understand the condition, they are likely to be supportive.

Q When should I become concerned about my attacks?

Since migraine can be a progressive illness you must prevent attacks if they become frequent. If you start experiencing more than 3 headache days a month, you must start a preventive migraine treatment program.

Q How can I prevent migraine attacks?

You can prevent migraine attacks by limiting or reducing the excitability of brain cells. Think of your brain as turning on a migraine attack. You always have the potential for having a migraine. A migraine treatment program is like a software program that filters an unwanted migraine attack. There are many ways to prevent attacks, all of which decrease the excitability of brain cells, thus reducing the brain's ability to start a migraine attack.

Q How do medications work to prevent migraine?

Medications used to prevent migraine attacks work in different ways. Some decrease the effect of epinephrine on brain cells, while others increase serotonin or function like serotonin. Treatment may be as simple as one medication, or involve a combination of medications. Eliminating as many triggers as possible reduces the potential for a migraine, and less medication is needed to reduce the likelihood of an attack. With time, many migraine sufferers are able to eliminate the need for medication once migraine frequency has decreased to fewer than 2 attacks per month.

Q So can I simply take a pill for my migraine?

Medication may stop your migraine. However, as effective as current medication treatment is today, it cannot prevent or treat every attack. The more frequently you experience attacks, the more likely it is that your migraine will get worse and that you will develop central sensitization (see p27). Avoidance of migraine triggers is an important part of your treatment program.

Q Why would I want to take a pill every day when I only have a migraine once in a while?

The objective in using migraine preventive medications is to help prevent migraine attacks and reduce the severity of an attack. Migraine is a progressive illness. If attacks occur more than once a week, the illness is likely to progress to chronic daily headache (more than 15 headache days a month). Preventive medications help augment the comprehensive migraine treatment program. You and your doctor can decide the best medication for your treatment based on the migraine or headache type, the severity and frequency of your attacks, additional illnesses that may be worsened or helped by the medication, and the presence of medication overuse headache (see pp78–81).

Q What if I have tried preventive medication and it did not work?

It is not uncommon for people with longstanding migraine to lose faith in preventative medications. They feel they have seen enough of doctors and pills. Many times the preventive medications were tried for too short a time, the dose was too high and caused side effects, or the migraine sufferer was still using medication aimed at stopping an attack that made the preventive medication ineffective. It is essential that migraine is not undertreated. You must not give up on preventive treatment because by doing so you risk developing chronic daily headache.

Q When do I need to take preventive migraine medication?

Starting a daily preventive medication depends on how well you are responding to your comprehensive treatment program. Lifestyle changes may reduce the frequency and severity of attacks without preventive medications. If migraine attacks last more than 2 hours and occur more than once a week, preventive medications are needed. Preventive medications can be stopped if you do not have a migraine for more than 8 months.

TAKING MEDICATION

Understanding how migraine medications work as part of your comprehensive treatment program to prevent migraine attacks is essential for your success. The following tips will help you get the most out of your preventive medications.

- Be realistic about what you think a medication can do for you.
- Understand how the medication helps prevent migraine attacks.
- Be aware of the potential side effects, both temporary and long-term.
- Understand which side effects mean you should to stop taking the drug.
- Know that all drugs have side effects; most disappear as medication is continued. Low doses taken initially and slowly raised have fewer side effects.
- Combine an aggressive nondrug treatment program to reduce migraine triggers with preventive medication for the best outcome.

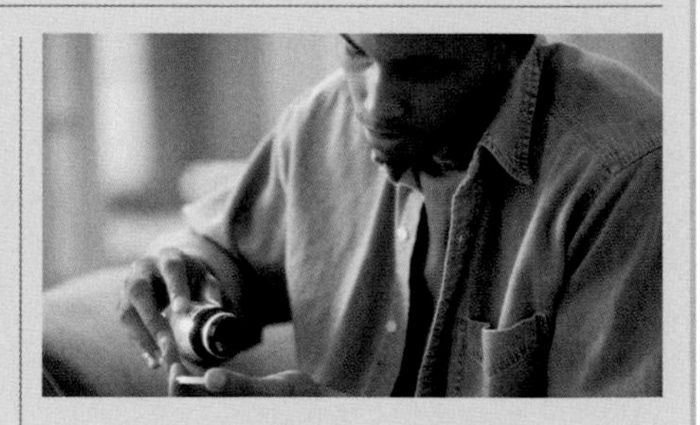

- Be aware that preventive migraine medications take 3–4 weeks to start working and should be used for 12 weeks at the correct dosage to see if the drug is effective.
- Remember that preventive medication will not work if you take any that cause medication overuse headache.

Q Can pills for high blood pressure (antihypertensives) prevent migraine?

Yes, beta-blockers and calcium channel blockers are types of antihypertensive medicines that can help prevent migraine. However, it is not understood exactly why these medications prevent migraine attacks.

Q What are beta-blockers?

Beta-blockers are medications used to block epinephrine. Although this group of medications has not been compared in formal studies to the other medications for preventing migraine, they are still some of the most effective medications for migraine prevention. The medications were initially used to treat hypertension (high blood pressure), but are now used in treating heart disease, heart rhythm problems, and anxiety. Only two of the medications have been studied thoroughly enough in the treatment of migraine so far to obtain approval from the US Food & Drug Administration (FDA).

Q How do doctors think beta-blockers may prevent migraine?

Beta-blockers work by blocking receptors for epinephrine, a chemical responsible for the "fight-or-flight" response. They may help prevent migraine by controlling the hyperactivity of the epinephrine system that occurs in people with migraine, but no studies have proven this.

Q What are the possible side effects of beta-blockers?

The possible side effects vary with each individual and the dose of the medication. The side effects may decrease or disappear with time and are less troublesome if the initial dose is low and then slowly increased, if needed. The possible side effects include fatigue, drowsiness, orthostatic hypotension (drop in blood pressure on standing), depressed mood, sexual dysfunction, exercise intolerance (tiring quickly during exercise), aggravation of asthma, weight gain, sleep disturbances, and vivid dreams.

Medications used for migraine prevention

No medications have been developed solely for the purpose of migraine prevention. However, medications used to treat other medical conditions have been found to prevent migraine. The main classes of medication used to prevent migraine are antihypertensives (used for high blood pressure), antidepressants (used for anxiety and depression), and anticonvulsants/neurostabilizers (used for epilepsy or seizures). Antihypertensives used for migraine may be either beta-blockers or calcium channel blockers. Antidepressants used for migraine may be

MIGRAINE PREVENTIVE MEDICATIONS

ANTIHYPERTENSIVES	USUAL EFFECTIVE DOSE (MG)	FDA APPROVED
Beta-blockers		
Propranolol	60–320	Yes
Timolol	20–60	Yes
Atenolol	50–200	No
Metoprolol	50–200	No
Nadolol	20–240	No
Calcium channel blocker		
Verapamil	80–360	No

ANTICONVULSANTS (NEUROSTABILIZERS)	USUAL EFFECTIVE DOSE (MG)	FDA APPROVED
Divalproex sodium	500–1,000	Yes
Topiramate	50–200	Yes
*Levetiracetam	750–3,000	No
Gabapentin	1,200–3,000	No
Lamotrigine	100–200	No
*Zonisamide	100–300	No

tricyclic, selective serotonin reuptake inhibitors (SSRIs), or serotonin and norepinephrine reuptake inhibitors (SNRIs). Some of these medications have undergone scientific study and are now approved by the Food & Drug Administration (FDA) to treat migraine. In the US, a medication does not have to be approved for a particular medical condition for it to be used to treat that disease; it only has to be approved for use in the US by the FDA.

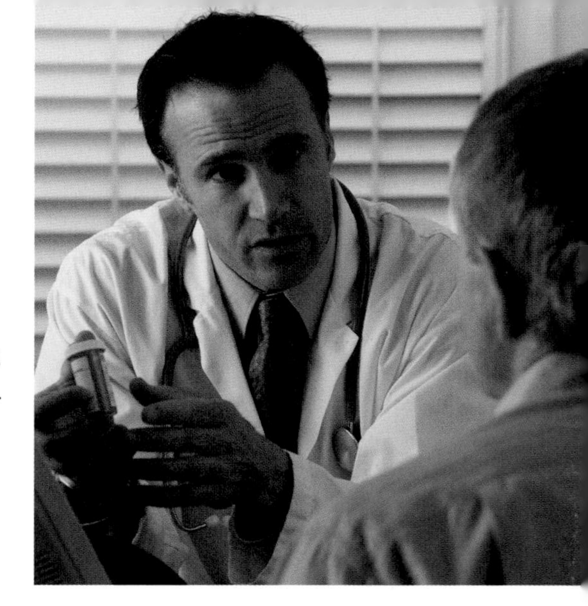

ANTIDEPRESSANTS	USUAL EFFECTIVE DOSE (MG)	FDA APPROVED
Tricyclic antidepressants		
Amitriptyline	25–150	No
Nortriptyline	25–150	No
Protriptyline	10–40	No
Doxepin	25–200	No
*Imipramine	25–150	No
Desipramine	25–150	No
Selective serotonin reuptake inhibitors (SSRIs)		
*Paroxetine	20–40	No
*Fluoxetine	20–40	No
*Escitalopram	10–40	No
*Sertraline	25–100	No
Serotonin and norepinephrine reuptake inhibitors (SNRIs)		
Venlafaxine	37.5–150	Yes
*Duloxetine	20–60	No

*Although these medications have been found helpful for migraine prevention, some specialists do not recommend routine use because scientific evidence is insufficient.

Q How do calcium channel blockers prevent migraine?

The electrical activity of brain cells occurs because substances called electrolytes cross the brain cell membranes much like a current in a battery. The tiny channels through which the electrolytes, such as sodium and chloride, flow are "gated" by calcium. The calcium channel blockers interact with this process and decrease the electrical activity. This interaction may be why these particular drugs help prevent migraine. The only calcium channel blocker available in the US that has been found to be somewhat helpful with migraine is verapamil. It is especially useful for basilar migraine, hemiplegic migraine, and migraine with aura (see Types of migraine, pp14–15).

Q What are the possible side effects of calcium channel blockers?

As with other medications, side effects vary with each individual and the dose. The possible side effects include fluid retention, sexual dysfunction, including decreased sperm motility (the ability of sperm to move or swim), constipation, weight gain, and heart block (interference with the heart's electrical conducting system).

Q How are antidepressants used for migraine prevention?

There are no large well-controlled studies that prove antidepressants help prevent migraine, so they have not been approved by the FDA for treatment of migraine. But many headache specialists find this group of drugs do help. It is assumed these drugs work by affecting serotonin (a brain communication chemical), much as they work for depression, anxiety, and other serotonin-related disorders. The types of antidepressant that are used for migraine prevention are tricyclic antidepressants, selective serotonin reuptake inhibitors (SSRIs), and serotonin and norepinephrine reuptake inhibitors (SNRIs).

Q What are the possible side effects of antidepressants?

The side effects of antidepressants vary, depending upon the dose and individuals. The possible side effects are sedation, weight gain, dry mouth, urinary retention, constipation, orthostatic hypotension (a sudden fall in blood pressure on standing), and sexual dysfunction.

Q How can medication used for epilepsy or seizures prevent migraine attacks?

Anticonvulsants (neurostabilizers) are medications used to prevent seizures. This group of medications has shown promise in treating migraine. It is not surprising that these medications work for migraine since, like epilepsy or a seizure disorder, migraine is cause by hyperexcitable brain cells. These medications work by stabilizing the electrical activity of brain cells, thus preventing a wave of excitation from spreading across the brain.

Q What are the possible side effects of anticonvulsants (neurostabilizers)?

The possible side effects of anticonvulsants can vary. These include fatigue or irritability, weight gain or weight loss, pins and needles sensation in the arms and legs, and swollen hands and feet. Most side effects are temporary; if they are intolerable, another medication can be used.

Q How will I know which medication is right for me?

It is important to discuss treatment options with your doctor. You can overlap your treatment of migraine with that of another medical problem. If you have high blood pressure, then beta-blockers may help treat both. In individuals with migraine and depression and/or anxiety, one of the antidepressants may help. However, if you have a problem that might be complicated by the medication, such as asthma with beta-blockers or weight gain with antidepressants, then an anticonvulsant such as topiramate may be the best choice.

Q What if I am sensitive to certain medications?

Sensitivity to some medications is not uncommon for people who have sought treatment for migraine. For many, the medication was started at a dose higher than they could tolerate, while others were not aware that certain side effects can go away with time or with a lower dose.

Q How can I avoid side effects as much as possible?

Some side effects are unavoidable. If a particular side effect is intolerable, you need to try a different medication. Most medications can be used successfully if the initial dose is small and gradual increases in dose are made slowly over time. Using a liquid, a sprinkle formulation, or a pill cutter can be very helpful in the beginning.

Q What if I tried a medication that was somewhat helpful but then the larger dose caused side effects?

Adding a second medication from a different group of preventive migraine medications may be helpful. This approach allows you to use two medications at a lower dose rather than one at a high dose, with consequent side effects. Maintaining an aggressive comprehensive treatment program that includes avoiding migraine triggers, regular exercise, and stress management should eliminate the need for excessive medication.

Q What if I forget to take a medication?

When you forget to take a medication, you may trigger a migraine attack or suffer from side effects, especially with antidepressants. It is important to take the medication as directed by your doctor. Initially, the medication will be more effective if you take regular pills twice a day. With better migraine control, you can change to the long-acting form called sustained release. Sustained release pills are usually taken only once a day and it is easier to remember to take them.

Q How can I remember to take my medication?

You can use a pill container with sections for each day of the week. But keep the medication out of the reach of children since most of these containers are not child-resistant. Taking your medication before a daily activity such as brushing your teeth, shaving, or showering may also be helpful. Some medications need to be taken at bedtime or after a meal, so check with your doctor for instructions regarding drug administration.

Q Will I have to take medication daily for the rest of my life?

Migraine differs from person to person. For most people with migraine, daily medication can be tapered off and eventually discontinued if migraine attacks drop to less than twice a month. The thought of stopping your daily medication should motivate you to treat your migraine with a comprehensive program. Once you have reduced the frequency of attacks, you should be able to maintain migraine control without daily medication if you continue to avoid triggers, reduce stress, and exercise regularly.

Q How long does it take for a preventive medication to start to "work?"

Preventive medications need at least a month to work once you have achieved an effective dose. Each medication will continue to become more effective over the succeeding 3 months. You cannot determine whether or not a medicine has been ineffective until you have taken it for 4 months.

Q How does one determine if the medication is "working?"

An effective preventive migraine medication needs to reduce the frequency, severity, and duration of your migraine attacks. A medication is deemed effective if it reduces frequency of migraine attacks by more than 50 percent. If the frequency of your migraine attacks has not been reduced by at least this amount, you need to change the treatment approach.

Other therapies for migraine

Q Are there other therapies that can work with preventive migraine medications?

There are several preventive complementary therapies for migraine. Some have been researched extensively and found to be effective; others have not been researched but have been used for years. The most recent preventive therapy, which is yet to be approved by the FDA, is the use of botulinum toxin (Botox) injections. Botox injections were used for years to treat muscle spasms in the face and neck. It was found that the treatment reduced the appearance of wrinkles, and it started to be used for cosmetic reasons. People with migraine began reporting an improvement in the frequency of their migraine attacks. Studies have shown mixed results on the effectiveness of Botox for the prevention of migraine attacks.

Q Should I consider getting Botox for my migraine?

As with many complementary therapies, Botox may not be that effective by itself, but when used with a comprehensive treatment program it may be helpful. It will not, however, cure your migraine. You may want to consider Botox injections if an effective trial of medications along with an aggressive comprehensive approach to your migraine treatment has failed to reduce the frequency of attacks. Botox injections can be expensive, and health insurance companies may or may not cover the treatment. My advice is that a better investment than Botox would be a treadmill to walk on everyday, as long as you use it and not allow it to become an expensive clothing rack.

Q What is a nerve block for migraine?

A nerve block is an injection of a local anesthetic around a nerve, causing an area to go numb. Occipital nerve block, for example, involves an injection around the occipital nerves in the scalp on the back part of the head. This procedure has not been well studied for the treatment of migraine.

Q How do trigger point injections help migraine?

Trigger point injections are used to help individuals with headache or with neck and upper back tightness or tension. Small amounts of salt water (saline) are injected with tiny needles into different areas of the tense or tight muscles. As with Botox injections, we do not know how this procedure helps prevent migraine; it may be more helpful if you just have frequent headaches. The procedure carries with it no real danger. However, before you make the financial investment it is important that you have treated your migraine aggressively with exercise, stress management, the reduction of as many triggers as possible, and the use of appropriate medication.

Q Can biofeedback or relaxation techniques be used to prevent migraine?

The use of a routine relaxation program is a very important part of your comprehensive migraine treatment program. The use of biofeedback for migraine prevention has been found to be very effective, especially in children. Whichever technique you decide to use, it needs to match your personality and belief system. You may want to experiment with different techniques until you find the one that brings you the most enjoyment and relaxation. It is very important that you maintain your relaxation routine. Relaxation techniques are very helpful, but only if you practice them regularly.

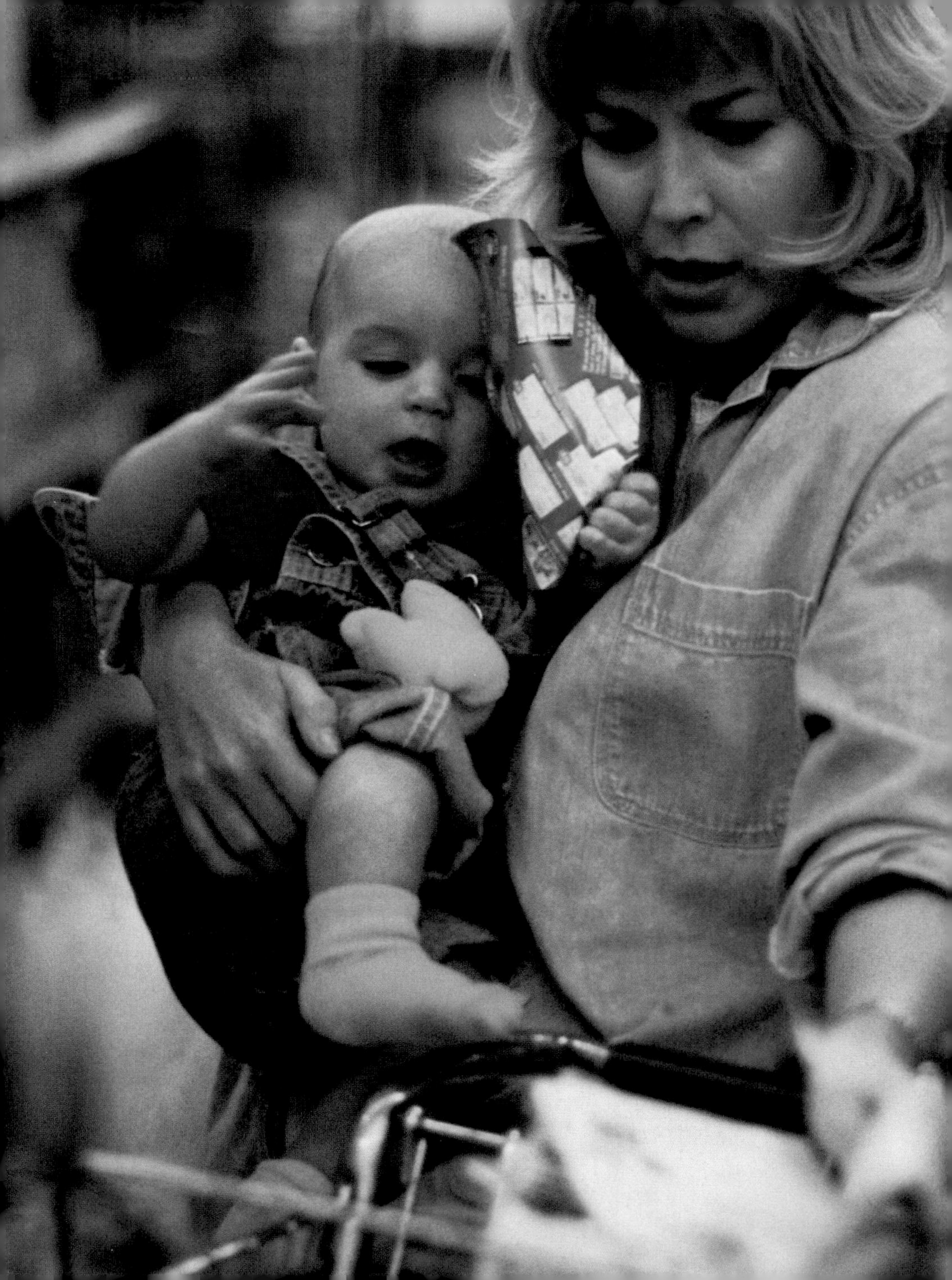

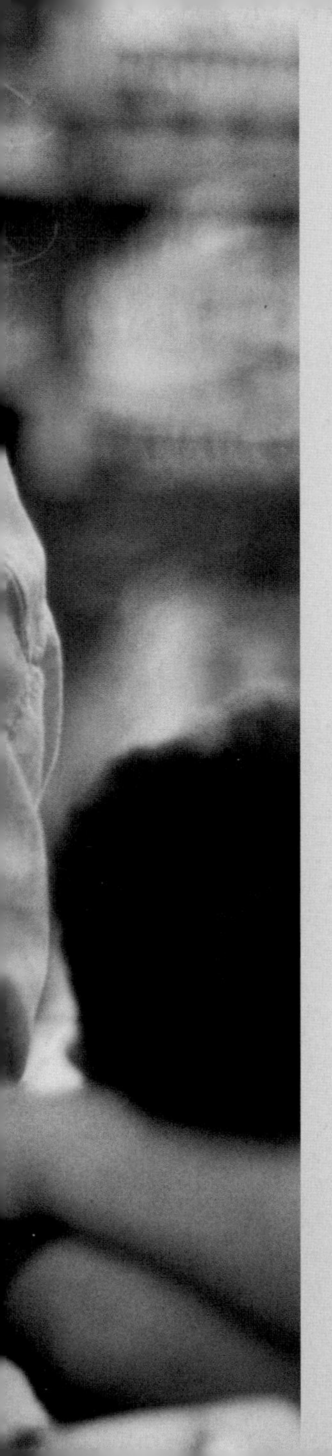

Migraine triggers

Your ability to identify and control migraine triggers plays a crucial role in checking migraine attacks. A migraine trigger excites brain cells and starts an attack. It can come from your external environment, such as food, or your internal environment, such as a change in hormone or blood sugar levels. Understanding how to control triggers with lifestyle adjustments is central to managing migraine.

Identifying migraine triggers

Q What are the triggers for migraine?

Many triggers can start a migraine attack. Any situation or substance can act to excite the brain cells of someone with migraine and trigger an attack. These range from stressful events and hormonal changes to drugs and changes in the weather (see box, right, for a detailed list).

Q How do migraine triggers cause an attack?

Migraine triggers cause hyperexcitable brain cells to become more excited by either acting directly on them or by increasing the level of epinephrine (a chemical that excites brain cells). Some scientists believe the triggers do not start the attack but simply intensify the symptoms of an attack already underway. Once the brain cells reach a certain level of excitation, an attack is triggered. Some studies have shown that the electrical reaction of the brain cells is more sensitive to a stimulus not only during an attack but also in between attacks.

Q What is the most common migraine trigger?

The most common trigger for a migraine attack is emotional stress. This is understandable since an emotionally stressful event or situation brings on what is called the "fight-or-flight" response. During such a response, epinephrine is released, which can hyperexcite brain cells and bring on an attack.

Q Is emotional stress the only thing that causes the "fight-or-flight" response?

No, the "fight-or-flight" response is the body's protective reaction to any thing or situation that threatens harm. "Stress" for the body could be, for example, low blood sugar or oxygen levels, low blood pressure, or any stress related to a medical illness.

Q Why do some things trigger a migraine attack in some people but not in others?

Triggers tend to vary among individuals. Many people with migraine can identify specific triggers while others have no idea. Some people know that they are more susceptible to one trigger than another. In some cases, several triggers work together to increase the likelihood of an attack. Each trigger affects the brain even if it doesn't lead to an attack; the closer triggers are to one another, the more likely it is that a migraine attack will occur. Often, a trigger is present hours to days before the attack but only when it combines with another trigger does it bring on a migraine attack.

Q Why do I need to identify and avoid triggers?

If you are able to identify and avoid or eliminate some of your triggers, you may be able to reduce the frequency of your attacks. Some studies have shown that trigger identification and avoidance can be as effective as daily preventative medications for migraine. Moreover, medications for migraine can become less effective if attacks occur too frequently.

RANGE OF MIGRAINE TRIGGERS

Migraine triggers may be internal (coming from inside you) or external (coming from your external environment). The list below gives some of the main triggers.

External triggers: Stressful events • Food/drink • Food additives • Schedule or time changes • Sleep disruption • Changes in eating habits • Weather change • Altitude change • Intense heat or cold • Intense light, sound, or odors • Overuse of certain medications • Drugs

Internal triggers: Hormonal changes, such as menstruation • Missing meals • Illness • Hypoglycemia (low blood sugar) • Dehydration

MIGRAINE AND THE STRESS RESPONSE

An appreciation of the "fight-or-flight" stress response helps you understand why certain situations trigger migraine attacks. During this response, epinephrine excites the hyperexcitable brain cells further, causing a migraine attack. Beta-blockers—drugs that block the effects of epinephrine—are very effective when used to prevent attacks.

Any situation that threatens the delicate balance of the body activates the stress response. This response prepares the body to react to the stressful stimulus, whether this is a physical threat, such as an attack by a wild animal, or an emotional stress, such as taking an exam.

Although the stress response is both vital and valuable, it can also be disruptive and damaging. The response, which evolved to prompt animals to fight or run away from harm, can be misplaced in human society. Humans rarely require the intense physical action generated by this response, yet our biology still provides it. When the stress response is activated repeatedly, it can have a harmful effect on the body. For some people, it can be a frequent trigger for migraine attacks.

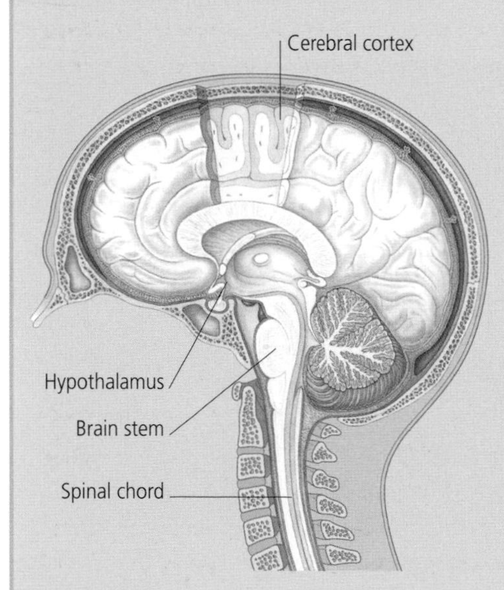

THE STRESS RESPONSE

During stressful situations, messages are carried along nerves from the cerebral cortex (where thought processes occur) to the hypothalamus. The hypothalamus activates autonomic nerves (nerves that carry information about automatic bodily processes) in the brain stem and prompts the release of epinephrine. This causes an increase in heart and breathing rates, blood pressure, and blood sugar levels, a slowing of the gastrointestinal tract, and dilation of the pupils. These changes prepare the body for fight or flight.

Internal triggers

Q How can menstruation and menopause trigger attacks?

During the last fortnight of the menstrual cycle, the level of estrogen (a female hormone) gradually decreases. This withdrawal directly affects brain cell function and can trigger a migraine attack. During menopause, a woman's body produces estrogen and progesterone (the sex hormones responsible for reproduction) more erratically. The disrupted estrogen can trigger migraine. Following menopause, estrogen and progesterone levels are consistently low, hence migraine can improve.

Q Why can missing a meal or eating too many carbohydrates cause an attack?

Missing a meal can lead to hypoglycemia (low blood sugar). It is thought that hypoglycemia triggers migraine by causing the release of epinephrine and other hormones associated with the stress response. These hormones lead to an increase in the blood sugar levels. The body then releases insulin to bring these levels down, which may fall too much. Eating too many carbohydrates has a similar effect, in addition to increasing blood sugar levels.

Q How does dehydration trigger a migraine attack?

The most likely explanation is the same as with hypoglycemia (see above). Any threat to the normal function of the brain and body can cause a stress response.

Q Why do I have a migraine attack when I stay up too late or sleep too late?

The body's biological cycles are regulated by the hypothalamus, which controls release of serotonin, which induces sleep, and epinephrine, which has an activating effect. In migraine, due to a disturbance in serotonin activity, epinephrine release is poor. This is the most likely reason why sleep disruption can trigger migraine.

Myth "Menstrual migraine is unavoidable"

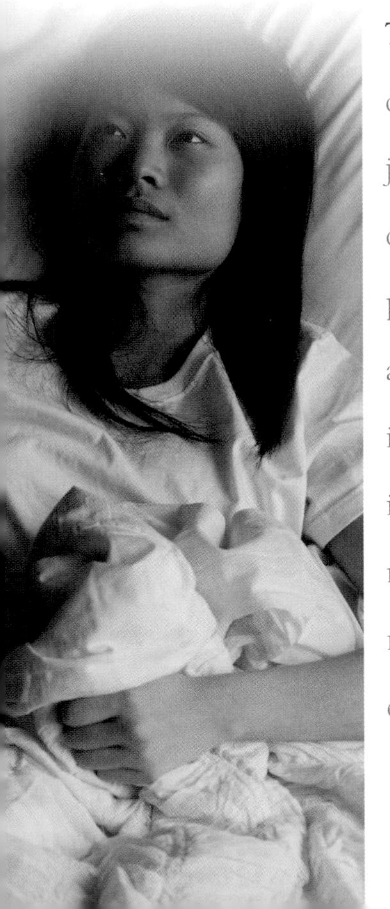

Truth Although menstrual migraine is the result of an internal trigger—the drop in estrogen levels just before menstruation—it is more likely to occur or to be more severe if other triggers are also present. Therefore, avoiding other triggers, such as sleep disturbance or missing a meal, is just as important for those with menstrual migraine as it is for anyone with migraine. By controlling the number of triggers present during the week before menstruation, menstrual migraine can be more easily treated or possibly avoided completely.

External triggers

Q Which foods and food additives can trigger a migraine attack?

As with other triggers, such as stress or menstruation, vulnerability to food triggers varies widely among individuals. The food triggers most commonly reported include wine, aged cheese, aged meats, caffeine, and citrus fruits. Others have been reported, but are not as widely accepted by experts. These include chocolate, aspartame, glutamate, and other food additives containing glutamate (for details, see pp70–73).

Q How do food and drink trigger migraine attacks?

Theories on how food or food additives trigger migraine vary considerably, with studies showing mixed results. Each food, food additive, or drink may act as a stimulant and excite brain cells, thus triggering an attack. Some food triggers may cause the release of epinephrine, triggering an attack indirectly, while others, such as glutamate, can act directly on brain cells, causing excitation.

Q What substances in a food or drink can trigger a migraine?

Various substances in food and beverages can trigger migraine. These include tyramine, phenylethylamine, monosodium glutamate, aspartame, and caffeine. Despite the lack of scientific evidence, many experts believe that avoiding these dietary chemicals may help reduce attacks. Most treatment programs advise avoiding alcohol, chocolate, matured cheese, wine, and monosodium glutamate (MSG). If you are finding it difficult to control your migraine, it may be worth trying a migraine-friendly diet for a few months. Once the attacks are well controlled, you can experiment with reintroducing specific foods or beverages, provided no other migraine triggers are present.

Food and drinks that may trigger migraine

Avoiding some of the common food and drink triggers may help prevent migraine attacks, especially during times of increased vulnerability. If you are experiencing frequent migraine attacks or other migraine triggers, such as stress or menstruation, then controlling migraine food and drink triggers can sometimes help you avoid or decrease the severity of an attack.

BEVERAGES

- Carob, chocolate, or cocoa
- Diet drinks (all contain aspartame)
- Energy drinks
- Flavored coffee/ creamers
- Lemon/lime sodas
- Liqueurs
- Malt beverages
- Sherry
- Sports drinks with fruit triggers
- Tea—all varieties
- Wine or beer (including those that are alcohol-free)

BREADS AND CEREALS

- All containing butylated hydroxyanisole (BHA), butylated hydroxytoluene (BHT), yeast extracts, or other additives
- Croutons (unless additive-free)
- Doughnuts (unless additive-free)
- Sour dough breads
- Stuffing mixes

DAIRY PRODUCTS

- Buttermilk
- Chocolate milk
- Skimmed milk
- Sour cream

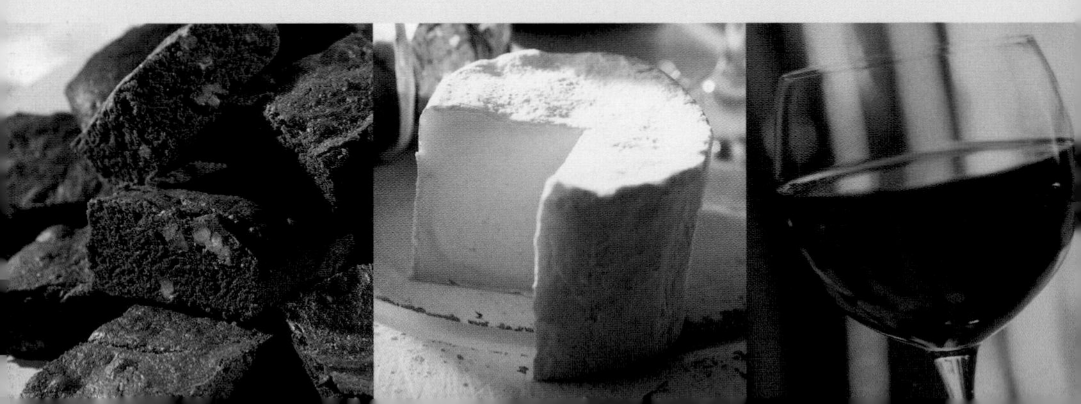

- Yogurt
- Aged cheeses including: blue; boursault; brie; brick; camembert; cheddar; feta; gouda; jack; mozzarella; muenster; parmesan; provolone; roquefort; romano; stilton; swiss

DESSERTS

- All containing aspartame
- All containing chocolate
- All containing fruit triggers (see below)
- All containing nuts
- Gelatin
- Licorice
- Maple syrup
- Molasses

FRUIT

- All over-ripe and dried fruit
- Avocados
- Bananas
- Cantaloupe
- Dates
- Figs
- Grapefruit
- Grapes
- Guava
- Honeydew melon
- Kiwis
- Lemons
- Limes
- Mangoes
- Nectarines
- Oranges
- Papayas
- Pineapples
- Plums
- Prunes
- Raisins
- Tangerines

MEATS AND FISH

- Any meat or fish that contains tenderizer, soy sauce, soy products, nitrates, or yeast extracts.
- Anchovies
- Caviar
- Corned beef
- Dried game meat
- Dried or canned ham
- Dried/salted fish
- Hot dogs
- Liver
- Meat extracts
- Packaged meats
- Pepperoni or salami
- Pickled herring
- Sardines
- Sausage (fermented, containing nitrates and/or nitrites)
- Snails
- Tuna containing vegetable broth

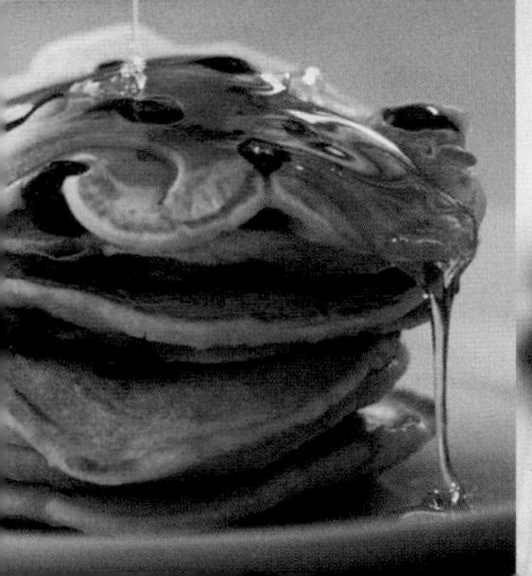

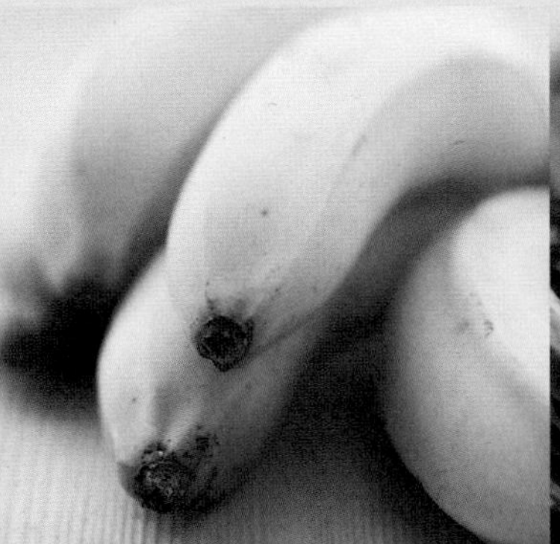

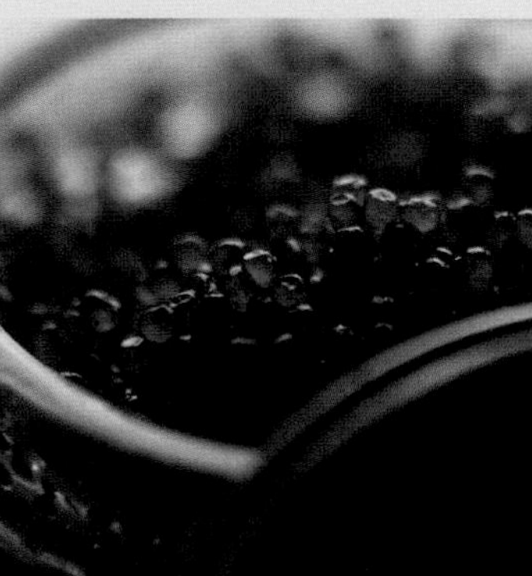

- Cured, fermented, pickled, or processed, smoked meats

NUTS AND SEEDS AND THEIR OILS

- All nuts
- Caraway seeds/oil
- Flax seeds/oil
- Peanut butter
- Peanuts/oil
- Poppy seeds/oil
- Pumpkin seeds/oil
- Sesame seeds/oil
- Sunflower seeds/oil

SAUCES, SOUPS, AND GRAVIES

- All bouillon cubes and soups
- All broth (except homemade)
- All canned and bottled gravies
- All canned and bottled soups
- All bottled sauces with monosodium glutamate
- Sauces such as sweet and sour, worcestershire, soy, and teriyaki sauce
- Ramen noodles
- Wine vinegar

VEGETABLES

- Beets
- Fava beans
- Garbanzo beans
- Italian beans
- Kidney beans
- Lentils
- Lima beans
- Mushrooms
- Navy beans
- Onions (except flakes and powder)
- Pickles
- Pea pods
- Pinto beans
- Pole or broad beans
- Rhubarb
- Sauerkraut

FOOD ADDITIVES

- Aspartame
- Autolyzed yeast
- Beef flavoring
- Butylated hydroxyanisole (BHA)
- Buylated hydroxytoluene (BHT)
- Carrageenan
- Caseinate
- Corn starch or modified corn starch
- Flavor(s) or flavoring(s)
- Gelatin
- Glutamate or glutamic acid
- Guar gum
- Hydrolyzed plant protein (HPP)

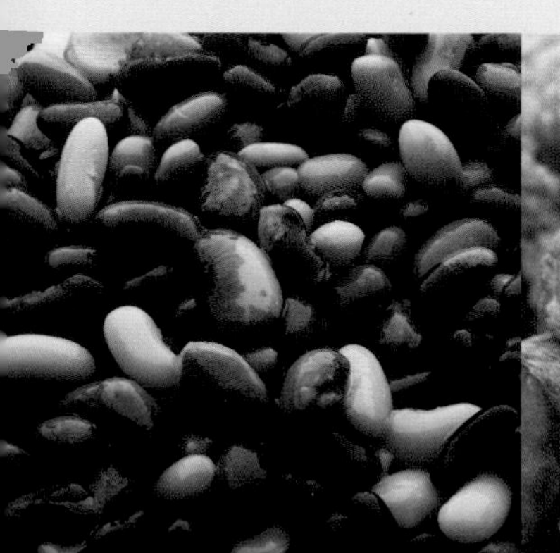
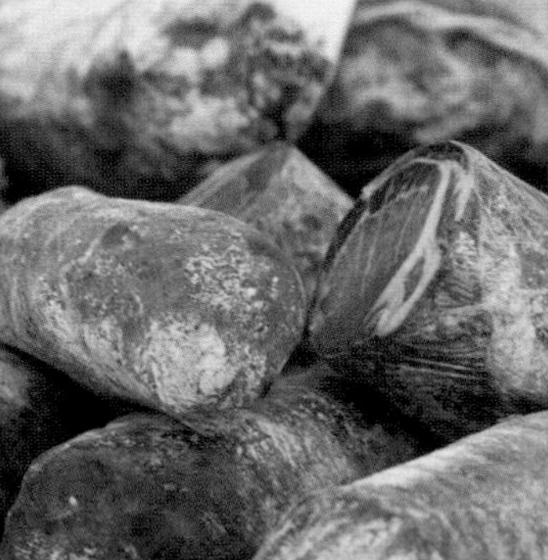
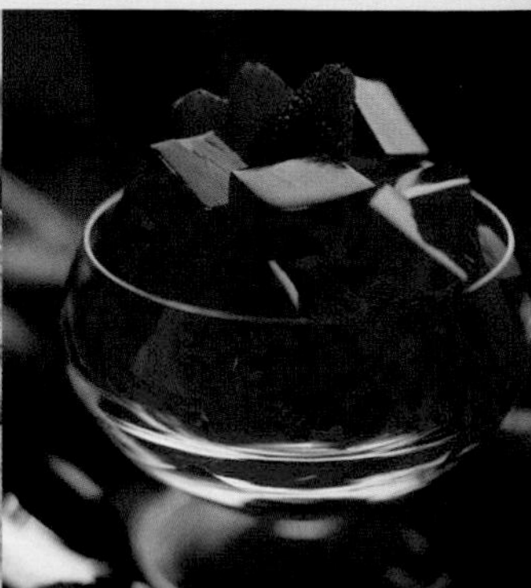

- Hydrolyzed soy protein
- Hydrolyzed vegetable protein (HVP)
- Kombu extract
- Malt: barley/extract/flavoring
- Maltoxdextran
- Modified food starch
- Monosodium glutamate (MSG)
- Natural flavoring
- Seasoned salts (unless contain spices without additives)
- Soy or soy products
- Soy lecithin
- Sulfites
- Smoke flavoring
- Seasoning(s)/salts
- Tenderizer
- Whey or whey protein
- Vegetable oil with soy
- Yeast extract

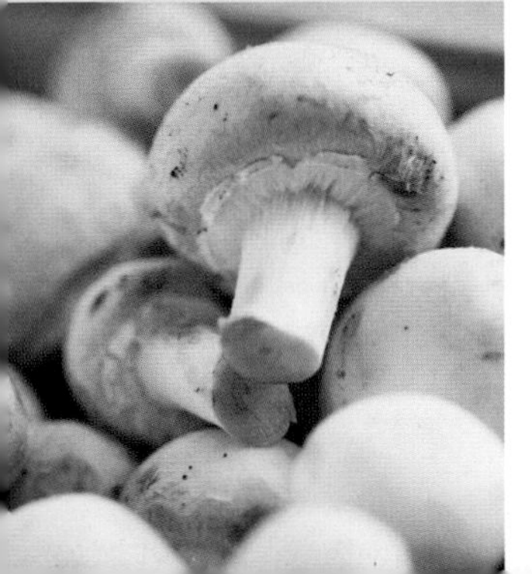

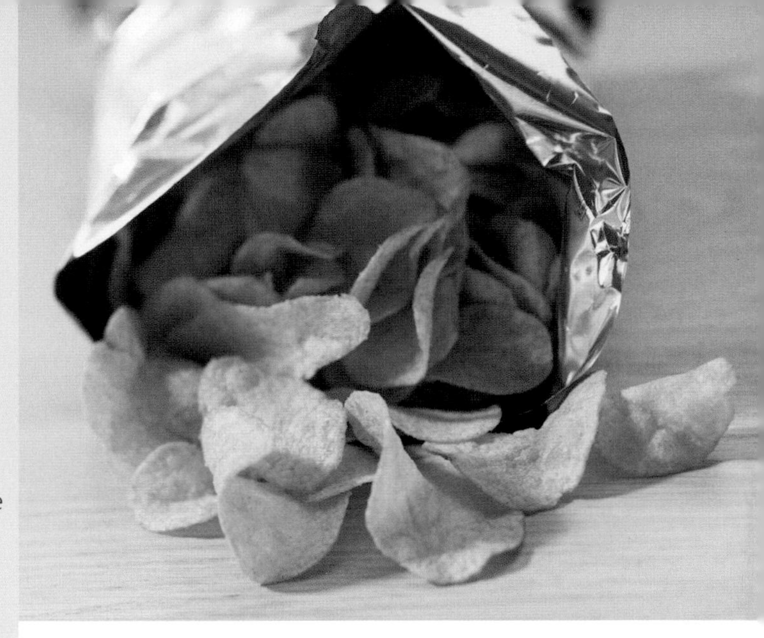

PACKAGED FOOD

Prepackaged food usually contains additives but not always. Check mints, toothpaste, sugarless gum, and any food with "sugarless" on the label, medications, and all diet and "low" fat foods for aspartame. Additives are often found in make-up, lipstick, and lotions as well.

The following packaged food may contain additives:

- Commercial salad dressings and mayonnaise
- Flavored potato chips
- Frozen foods (lunch or dinner entrees)
- Health bars and drinks
- Multivitamins
- Packaged or frozen meals
- Pizza (commercial)
- Pickled, preserved, or marinated food
- Protein powders (unless rice or egg protein only)
- Weight loss powders
- Weight loss prepared foods and supplements
- Bottled sauces (with aspartame, MSG, soy)

Q How can a change in my schedule, sleep patterns, or eating habits trigger a migraine attack?

The cells in your body need to be maintained in stable, constant conditions. Any change in your external or internal environment requires that the body makes adjustments in its physiology (biological functions). Unexpected variations in your schedule, sleep patterns, or eating habits require such adjustments. All of these situations have been found to trigger migraine attacks. It is not well understood why, but it is recognized that people with migraine benefit from following strict routines. Further, the use of medications to prevent attacks can raise the threshold and help people with migraine to be less vulnerable to these triggers.

Q Why do I have migraine attacks during or after a stressful event?

Emotional stress triggers an attack because it leads to the "fight-or-flight" response. The cause of stress varies among individuals. What may seem very stressful to one person may be a mere aggravation for another. The important point is that emotional stress is the most commonly reported trigger for a migraine attack. Reducing stress is very important for the successful treatment of migraine.

Q Why do I often have a migraine attack on weekends?

Many people with migraine can get through a busy or stressful week without an attack, only to experience one when everything calms down. The stressful situation may have passed, but the biological changes caused by it continue. For those with migraine, the genetic problem with serotonin (a "calming" brain chemical) makes it difficult for the brain to decrease the excitation caused by epinephrine released during the stress response. Stress, like other migraine triggers, may need to be present for a few days before it causes the brain cells to be excited enough to trigger a migraine attack.

Q How can weather and altitude changes trigger an attack?

Although migraine attacks are frequently triggered by weather and altitude changes, we do not know why. Migraine attacks may occur because the body needs to make adjustments in physiology related to changes in atmospheric pressure.

Q Why do I get a migraine attack when I travel?

Travel is often associated with several migraine triggers in the same time period. For example, the time zone may change or the travel may lead to a change in eating habits or in sleep patterns, so it is not surprising that migraine attacks occur while traveling. All these changes can trigger attacks because they require that the body makes adjustments to its biological functions.

Q How do some odors, bright light, or loud noise trigger migraine attacks?

It is not well understood why odors, bright light, or noise may trigger a migraine. We do know that the brain is very sensitive to input from the body's senses. Since the brain cells of those with migraine are thought to be hyperexcitable, an exaggerated reaction to sensory input is a possible explanation.

Q Does the environment trigger an attack or am I only sensitive to environmental changes because I am having a migraine attack?

This is an excellent question—unfortunately, no one knows for certain. We do know that an attack can be triggered by a visual stimulus, because this method has been used to study migraine. But it does also appear that the better you control migraine the less sensitive you will be to triggers. It is important that you treat the illness so that you do not find yourself living in an environmental bubble, fearful that a trigger is lurking around every corner. On the other hand, it is also important to identity factors in your environment that can trigger migraine and try to avoid them as much as possible.

Q How do medications trigger attacks?

The overuse of certain medications, especially those used to stop migraine attacks, can also trigger more attacks. Medications for other illnesses may also trigger migraine. Many over-the-counter drugs and "natural" herbal remedies cause medication overuse headaches, while others simply trigger an attack because they are stimulants. It is important to reduce or eliminate any medication that increases the frequency of headaches.

Q How can "natural" herbal supplements trigger headaches?

Many "natural" supplements used for weight loss or fatigue contain caffeine or "caffeinelike" chemicals and are stimulants. Any stimulant can increase the level of epinephrine in the blood and brain, as does stress or certain foods and beverages. To avoid repeated migraine attacks, you must avoid as many triggers as possible, including "natural" stimulants.

Q Does smoking trigger migraine?

Smoking (or using nicotine in other forms, such as chewing tobacco or snuff) may trigger migraine and those addicted to smoking should quit. You can expect some withdrawal headaches when you first stop using nicotine but these will clear up with time. Even if you are not a smoker yourself, you still need to avoid exposure to second-hand smoke.

Q How does smoking or the use of nicotine trigger migraine attacks?

Nicotine affects the brain cells in 2 ways. For a short time it acts as a stimulant, then, within a few minutes, it has a sedative effect. By stimulating brain cells, nicotine can act as a trigger. Subsequently, once its level in the blood drops, the withdrawal of its sedative effect can also trigger an attack. Additionally, cigarettes contain other chemicals that could trigger a migraine attack.

Q Can the use of recreational drugs worsen migraine?

Recreational drugs are harmful for several reasons, but stimulants such as cocaine and methamphetamine can cause a stroke in those with migraine. More sedative drugs, such as marijuana and heroin, can cause medication overuse headaches, as can prescription narcotics, such as codeine and hydrocodone, and anti-anxiety drugs, such as diazepam or alprazolam.

Q Does the use of recreational drugs do more than trigger a migraine?

Stimulants such as methamphetamine, cocaine, and ecstasy not only overstimulate the epinephrine chemistry of the brain but damage the serotonin system as well. Serotonin not only prevents a migraine attack but also balances the functions of epinephrine and dopamine in the brain. Dopamine, like epinephrine, excites brain cells. For example, people with schizophrenia have increased dopamine levels as well as severe intractable headaches. Excessive use of cocaine, ecstasy, or methamphetamine increases dopamine levels, causing drug-induced, schizophrenic-like symptoms.

Q How do sedative drugs trigger migraine attacks?

Drugs that sedate, including alcohol, do so by decreasing the excitability of brain cells. These drugs typically have a direct effect on brain cell receptors that are usually used by brain chemicals (neurotransmitters) that are naturally calming. The continued use of sedative drugs causes the brain to be less responsive to these neurotransmitters. When the drug is no longer present in the body, the brain is unable to decrease brain cell excitability, which then leads to a drug withdrawal headache. The same mechanism causes medication overuse headache when medications that stop migraine attacks are used too frequently.

Medication overuse headache

Q Can my medication give me a headache?

Yes, there are medications that, taken on a routine basis, can cause a headache known as medication overuse headache (previously called rebound headache). Some medications are known to induce headaches, while the effects of others remain controversial. It is important that you do not use any migraine-relief medication for more than 2 days a week. Therefore, an aggressive preventive treatment program is essential.

Q Why do I need to be concerned about medication overuse headache?

In headache clinics in the US, nearly 80 percent of patients with chronic daily headache (more than 15 headache days per month) have medication overuse headache. If you are among the millions whose headaches have become chronic, you probably have medication overuse headache in addition to your main headache disorder.

Q What are the symptoms of medication overuse headache?

The daily headaches may vary depending upon the type of medication that is being overused. Those caused by the excessive use of analgesics resemble tension headaches, whereas triptan (see p128) overuse headaches are more like migraine headaches. The headaches caused by medication become more frequent over time, causing the user to become dependent upon the medication. This is not an addiction, but it is a dependency because if you do not take the pill, you get a severe headache. The more you take the pills, the more headaches you have, and the more pills you need to take.

Q How do I avoid medication overuse headache?

Taking a medication for a headache for more than 3 days a week can cause medication overuse headache. A treatment program that includes effective therapy to stop migraine attacks without the overuse of medications is essential for the control of migraine. If migraine attacks are occurring more than 3–4 times a month, then preventive medication may be needed. Daily medications do not have to be taken forever. Once you reduce the frequency of migraine to less than 2 attacks a month, you can slowly reduce the preventive medication.

Q Could a certain medication that I am taking for another problem cause medication overuse headache?

Yes, frequent use of analgesics for any type of pain can cause medication overuse headaches in individuals with migraine. Many people with medication overuse headache think their headaches have a different cause. For example, they may believe that their headache is due to a sinus problem or an allergy because many of the medications used to treat sinus congestion and allergic symptoms can cause medication overuse headache. In fact, sinus or allergy problems do not cause a chronic daily headache; it is the medication used for the sinus symptoms or allergy. Stopping the overused medications brings a significant reduction in the frequency of headaches.

Q Apart from chronic daily headache, are there other problems associated with medication overuse?

Yes. You may develop a dependence on symptomatic medication, and medications for preventing migraine may become less effective. If you are overusing a medication and consequently the associated migraine symptoms of nausea and sensitivity to light or sound are less severe and less frequent than during typical migraine, you may not be diagnosed with migraine and may therefore not receive appropriate treatment.

Q Why do some drugs cause medication overuse headache?

Experts do not know why medication overuse headache develops in those who have migraine. Theories vary from a change in neurotransmitter function to a "rewiring" of the pain control system in the brain. What we do know is that by stopping the offending medication, daily headaches stop and migraine preventive medication is more effective.

MEDICATIONS THAT CAN CAUSE MEDICATION OVERUSE HEADACHE

Many different medications can be associated with medication overuse headache. Some of these are prescription, some over-the-counter (nonprescription), and some are considered natural herbal medications. Medications containing analgesics are the most common cause of medication overuse headache. These painkillers range from acetaminophen, found in nearly every over-the-counter medication, to very addictive opioids (narcotics).

- Acetaminophen
- Combinations of acetaminophen, aspirin, and caffeine
- Combinations of acetaminophen or aspirin and butalbital plus caffeine, with or without codeine
- All sinus/cold pills, nasal sprays, eye drops (unless pure steroid or pure antihistamine)
- All opioid (narcotic) painkillers (codeine)
- All sedatives (sleeping pills)
- All antianxiety medications
- All hypnotics (sleeping pills)
- All muscle relaxants (except baclofen)
- Herbal energy or diet pills

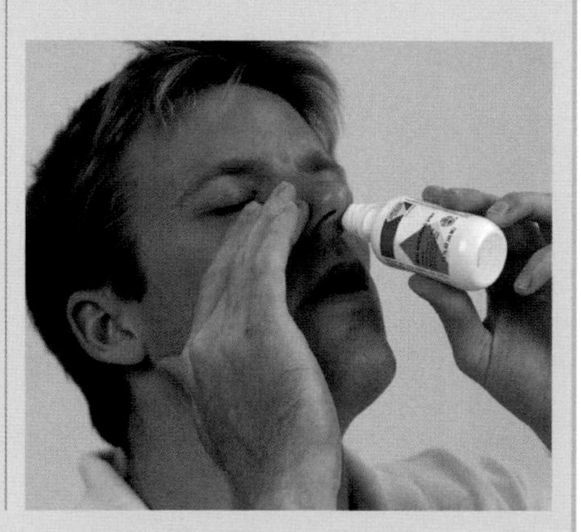

Q What should I do if I think my headache is due to medication overuse?

The first step to treating any headache problem is getting the right diagnosis so, if you have headaches that trouble you, you should see a doctor. Once you have been diagnosed with migraine, it is important that you avoid the overuse of any medication that could complicate your treatment. For those who are experiencing medication overuse headache, it is imperative to treat the underlying migraine, as well as the overuse headache. Suddenly stopping medications can cause withdrawal headaches unless you and your doctor plan ahead. Failure to maintain control of the headaches can convince you that the only way out is to return to using the pills that have complicated your problem. For the best results, see a doctor who is familiar with the treatment of medication overuse headache. Some individuals may require the expertise of a headache specialist. However, do not give up—migraine and headache disorders are treatable. No one should be told to just go home and live with the pain.

Q Can a medication cause a headache that is not a rebound headache?

Yes, there are medications used for other health problems that may have headache as a side effect.and may trigger migraine attacks. The medications that are most likely to trigger migraine are those that widen blood vessels, such as those used for angina, high blood pressure, and sexual dysfunction. Some medications used for ulcer disease and certain antibiotics may aggravate migraine as well. Hormonal therapy with cyclical progestogen can trigger migraines too. If your migraine attacks increase in frequency after you start a new medication, or if you have difficulty controlling your migraine, you may need to investigate the possibility that another medication you are taking is interfering with your migraine control.

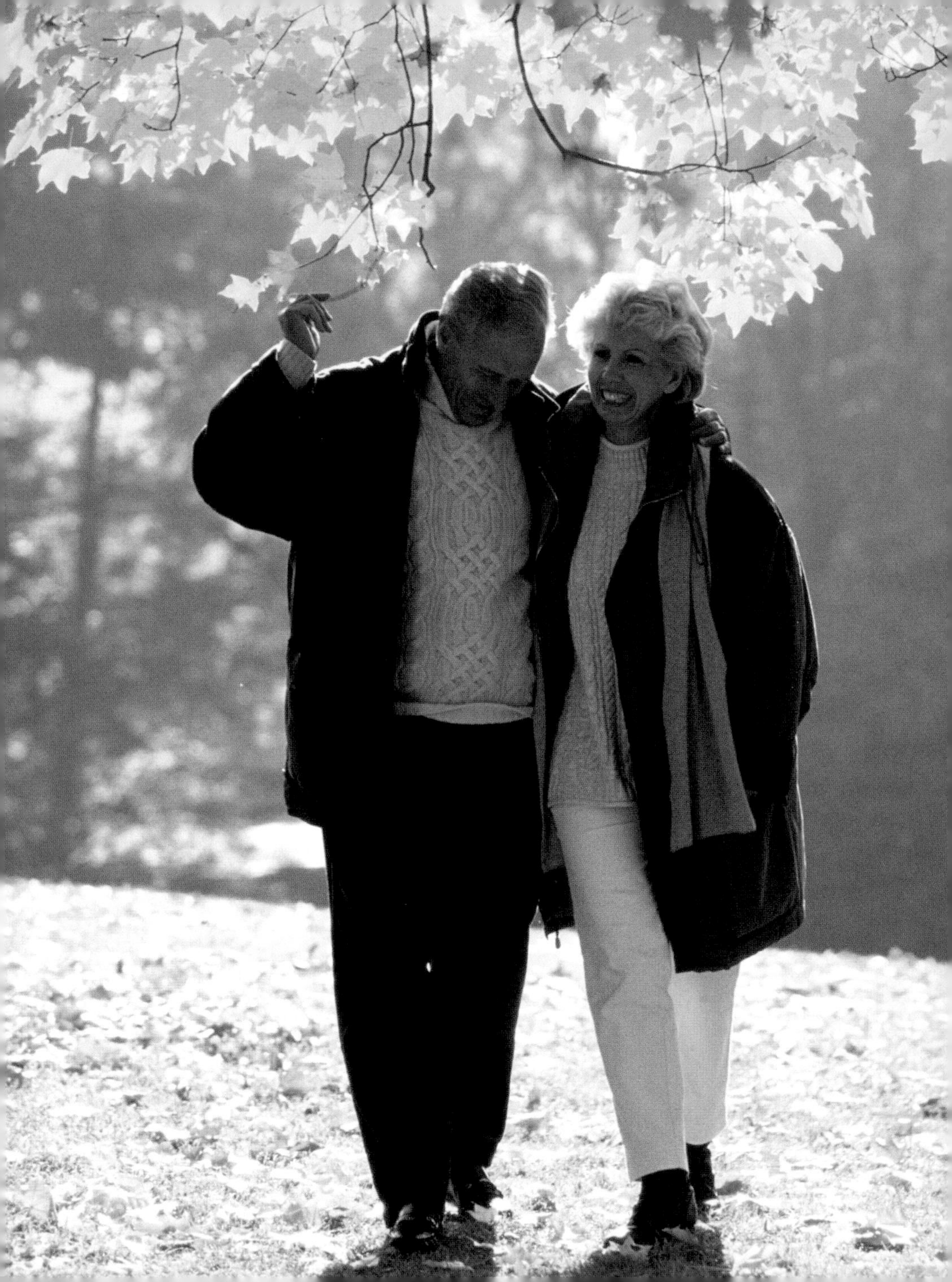

Making lifestyle changes

Accommodating necessary lifestyle changes of a successful treatment program requires planning and dedication. Once you start controlling your attacks, however, the new behavior will reinforce itself. Take it one day at a time. The joy of living your life without being at the mercy of migraine is worth the time and energy invested in a "migraine-friendly" lifestyle.

Migraine diary

Q Why should I keep a migraine diary?

Keeping a diary will help you avoid migraine triggers and maintain a consistent treatment program. Tracking your activities and noting when you have a migraine attack enables you to identify triggers, such as missed meals, traveling, stressful situations, or certain foods, and to avoid them as much as possible in future. Your diary also allows you to plan times for relaxation or stress management techniques as well as for exercise, and will help you stay dedicated to your treatment program.

Q How will the diary help me control the migraine attacks?

A diary will give you an accurate assessment of how well you are controlling your migraine. Most people experience periods of time when they get more frequent attacks, which can be very discouraging. It is very easy to give up during difficult times if you cannot see signs of immediate improvement. Looking back on times of better migraine control provides perspective and encourages you to persist with your treatment program, especially with changes in your lifestyle.

Q How can changing my lifestyle help my migraine?

Living a "migraine-friendly" lifestyle by avoiding triggers will not only lessen the frequency of attacks but may reduce and often eliminate the need for daily preventive medication. Most preventive medications are more effective if combined with lifestyle changes. As with many chronic conditions, lifestyle changes are at the heart of how well you manage the condition. It is important to understand that you must reduce triggers to prevent future migraine attacks, and not simply to avoid a single attack.

Q What if I am convinced my migraine is simply caused by stress?

Blaming only stress without seeing how the other triggers contribute to the frequency of your migraine attacks can make your migraine more difficult to treat successfully. You will come to view migraine attacks as inevitable during times of stress and may fail to take action that could prevent the attacks. During periods of stress, you can often eliminate or control other triggers and therefore prevent the attack while you are dealing with the stressful situation. Moreover, the migraine attack may be making you more prone to feeling stressed rather than the other way around and may have actually been triggered by something else.

Q I am reluctant to change my lifestyle. Do I really have to?

Many people with migraine feel the same as you. In the beginning, it is hard to believe that your migraine has anything to do with your diet or lifestyle. However, patients who take a comprehensive approach to their migraine treatment by avoiding as many triggers as possible usually find that the reduction in the frequency of their attacks is well worth all the hard work.

Q Why is it helpful to write down what I am eating or drinking?

Dietary changes for the successful treatment of migraine can be one of the most difficult challenges you will face. Some people may have more difficulty with dietary changes than others. Keeping track of what you are eating will help you alter your eating habits. Many people with migraine do not realize how many triggers are in the food they eat until they start writing down what they are eating. Unless you write down a list of what you eat and how you are eating, such as whether you miss meals, it can be difficult to see how your eating habits influence the frequency of the migraine attacks.

Keeping a migraine diary

Each day, write down in your diary all of the migraine triggers that may have occurred that day. Write down what you ate and when. Highlight each food or drink that you suspect is a trigger. The suggested format for your diary includes symbols to remind you what food groups you need to include with each meal; the number of symbols shows how many portions you should have. The symbols are: ♦ protein; ★ limited carbohydrate; ♥ free carbohydrates (see Menu planning, pp90–93). In the beginning, it is important to avoid as many of the food triggers as possible. You should also include in your diary the amount of exercise and relaxation time you have each day. It is helpful

HOW DO I RECORD MY MIGRAINE ATTACKS?

I recommend tracking migraine attacks with the identified triggers each day. The headache severity scale used in headache research is the most helpful way to rate headaches. With this scale, attacks are scored according to the level of disability. Headaches are rated on a 0–3 scale with 0 being headache-free and 3 a headache that prevents all activity.

TRIGGERS

A: Menstruation
B: Medical illness
C: Missing a meal
D: Too many carbohydrates
E: Dehydration
F: Stressful event
G: Food and drink
H: Schedule change or change in time
I: Sleep disruption
J: Change in eating habits
K: Weather change
L: Altitude change
M: Intense light, sound, or odors
N: Overuse of medications
O: Other medications

HEADACHE DISABILITY

0: No headache
1: Headache with no effect on activity
2: Headache interferes with activity
3: Headache inhibits or stops all activity

to document migraine attacks on a calendar with every month on a single page. You can circle the day of an attack with a different color corresponding to the headache severity scale. This allows you to examine trends related to the frequency of your migraine attacks and make improvements in your migraine control.

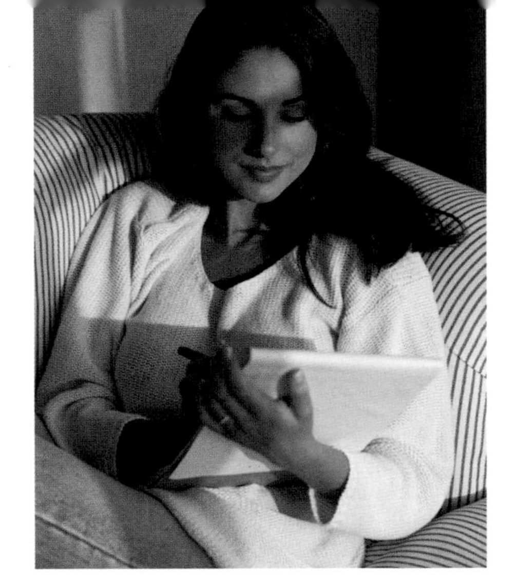

MIGRAINE DIARY

	Sun	Mon	Tues	Wed	Thurs	Fri	Sat
Breakfast ♦							
Snack ♦ ★½ ♥							
Lunch ♦♦ ★★ ♥♥							
Snack ♦ ★½							
Dinner ♦♦ ★★ ♥♥ (No carbs. after 6pm)							
Snack ♦ ★½							
Headache: 0-1-2-3 Triggers: (A-0)							
Exercise No. of min.							
Relaxation No. of min.							

Changing your eating habits

Q How long should I avoid possible food triggers?

Many foods are possible triggers for migraine. Each food that is a trigger contains a natural or artificial substance that can act as a stimulant, such as caffeine. To get the best results from your treatment program, I suggest you avoid all food and drink triggers until you experience fewer than 2 migraine attacks a month lasting less than 2 hours for at least 8 months. To find out which foods and drinks can trigger a migraine, see pp70–73.

Q What can I eat?

Those foods and drinks that are allowed (see pp91–93) are not triggers unless they contain food additives. You must read the labels on all commercial or packaged food and drink. It is important that you avoid hypoglycemia (low blood sugar levels) by not going too long without eating, and also that you do not eat too many carbohydrates with a high glycemic index (which raise blood sugar quickly). Such carbohydrates need to be limited and eaten along with a protein source. Carbohydrates with a high glycemic index are designated by the symbol ★ on the allowed food and drink list.

Q How do I change my eating habits to help control my migraine?

Planning is vital. Most of us are busy and eating on the run is common but eating prepackaged food and skipping meals will get you into trouble because of the additives in packaged food and low blood sugar that occurs if you don't eat regularly. Menu planning, shopping for "migraine-friendly" food, and preparing food takes perseverance. Sticking with it will be worth all your efforts because you will save time by not having a migraine.

Q How do I get started with a "migraine-friendly" diet?

The first step is to jot down in your migraine diary what you are eating and drinking. You cannot change your diet if you do not know how you are eating now. You may be surprised to know how many migraine triggers there are in what you eat and the way you eat it. Once you list your current diet, review the list of triggers. Plan to avoid as many as possible until you have control of your migraine.

Q How do I go about menu planning?

You can refer to the menu planning guide (see Menu planning, pp90–93) to help you reduce or eliminate potential migraine triggers. This menu plan also helps you to avoid hypoglycemia and dehydration. Consult your doctor first to make sure there are no reasons for you not to follow a "migraine-friendly" diet.

Q How do I find food without additives?

Buy as much fresh food as possible. If you think fresh food might have additives (for example, bakery bread often has preservatives), ask the store management. When buying packaged food, check the ingredients against the list of food and drink triggers (see pp70–73) to find out if it contains additives that should be avoided. Additive-free food is becoming increasingly popular nowadays.

Q Why is it so important that I limit certain carbohydrates?

There are a couple of reasons. First, eating carbohydrates with a high glycemic index (see Menu planning, pp90–93) causes a rapid release of insulin, leading to a drop in blood sugar that triggers a migraine attack. By decreasing such carbohydrates, you decrease the carbohydrate load and avoid hypoglycemia. The other reason is that excessive consumption of certain carbohydrates can lead to weight gain. Studies have shown that there is a correlation between obesity and the development of chronic migraine.

Menu planning

The list of allowed food and drinks (pp91–93) has a symbol by each food group to show if it is a protein (♦), a limited carbohydrate (★), or a free carbohydrate (♥). Limited carbohydrates are those with high glycemic index. The glycemic index is a ranking of carbohydrate-containing foods based on how fast they make blood sugar (glucose) levels rise. The higher the glycemic index, the faster a food will increase your blood sugar, with pure glucose having a rating of 100. Carbohydrates with a high glycemic index should be limited and eaten along with a protein source. These symbols are also used in the Migraine diary (see pp86–87) to help with menu planning and remind you to have a protein with each serving of limited carbohydrate.

When planning your menu, you must make sure you have adequate protein intake to avoid headaches. Avoid all carbohydrates at breakfast and for your bedtime snack. It is critical that you drink at least 8 fluid ounces of water with each meal and snack. You must eat every 3 hours while awake. Remember, the in-between meal snacks are just that, a snack. You are not eating because you are hungry; you are eating to control your headaches. Do not exceed 5 servings (100 grams) of limited carbohydrates per meal. Eating more than 100 grams of limited carbohydrate may trigger headaches by causing a drop in your blood sugar. You may need to increase the amount of limited carbohydrates to cope with increased physical activity or excessive weight loss.

Those with special dietary needs should consult a doctor before making any dietary changes.

- From the list of allowed foods, choose 5–6 servings of protein (♦). You need to have one serving for each meal and ½ serving for each snack.
- From the list of allowed foods choose 5 servings of limited carbohydrates (★), no more than 20 grams per serving; try for less. You may have these servings at any time except at breakfast and for a bedtime snack. Every serving of limited carbohydrate must be eaten with a serving of protein.
- You are allowed as many servings of free carbohydrates (♥)—vegetables—as you want. You need at least 5 servings a day for a healthy diet.

ALLOWED FOOD AND DRINK

Key to symbols: ♦ = protein ★ = limited carbohydrates ♥ = free carbohydrates

★ BEVERAGES

- Apple and pear juice
- Colas (no diet colas and only one serving of caffeine per day)
- Cranberry juice
- Cream soda
- Ginger ale
- Raspberry soda
- Strawberry juice
- Water

★ BREADS AND GRAINS

(no soy oil, soy additives, BHA/BHT)

- Bagels
- Corn tortillas
- English muffins
- Flour tortillas
- French bread
- French rolls
- Hamburger buns
- Italian bread
- Muffins
- Pita bread
- Rye bread
- Wheat and white bread

★ CEREALS, CRACKERS, AND COOKIES

(without any soy or vegetable oil)

- All cereals (without any additives or food triggers)
- Cream of rice and wheat
- Old-fashioned oatmeal
- Pretzels
- Rice cakes
- Rye crackers
- Tortilla corn chips

★ DRESSINGS, SAUCES, JAMS, AND VINEGAR

(no additives)

- Apple sauce
- Chili sauce
- Cranberry sauce
- Fruit jelly (allowed fruit)
- Jams (allowed fruit)
- Ketchup
- Mustard
- Pizza sauce

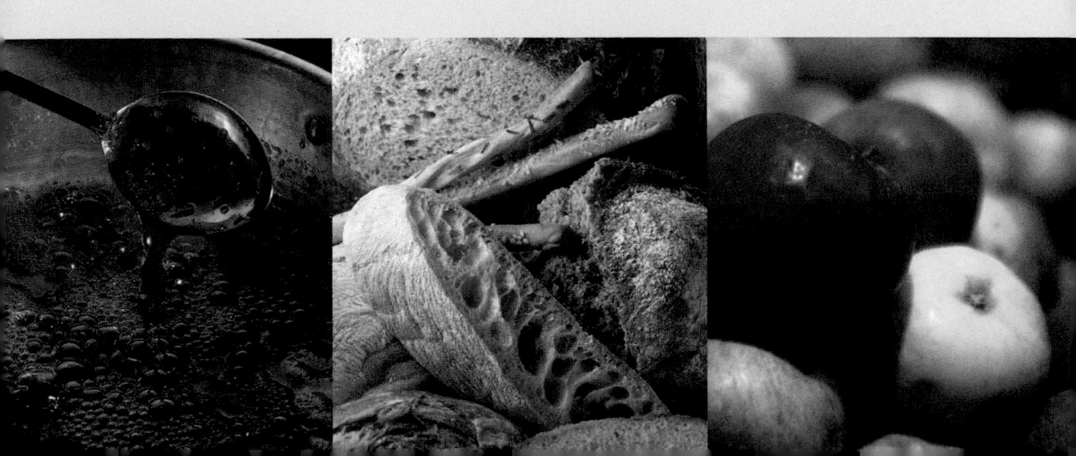

★ FRESH FRUIT

- Apples and pears
- Apricots
- Blueberries
- Canned or Dried (no sulfites or monosodium glutamate)
- Cherries
- Coconuts
- Cranberries
- Peaches
- Raspberries
- Strawberries
- Watermelons

★ TREATS

(limited quantity)

- Angel food cake
- Butterscotch chips
- Butterscotch pudding
- Carrots
- Corn
- Ice cream
- Pastas
- Peas
- Popcorn
- Potatoes
- Pound cake
- Rice (brown, white, or wild)
- Rice pudding
- Sugar
- Vanilla chips
- Vanilla pudding
- White cake mix

♦ DAIRY PRODUCTS

- American cheese
- Butter
- Cottage cheese
- Cream cheese
- Eggs
- Evaporated milk
- Farmer's cheese
- Fresh mozzarella
- Goat cheese, if not aged
- Heavy cream
- Margarine (additive-free)
- Milk (additive-free)
- Ricotta

♦ MEATS, POULTRY, AND SEAFOOD

(no additives)

- Beef
- Canned chicken
- Chicken
- Crab
- Deli meats (chicken, roast beef, turkey without MSG and nitrates)
- Fish
- Fresh pork (no bacon or ham)
- Lamb
- Lobster

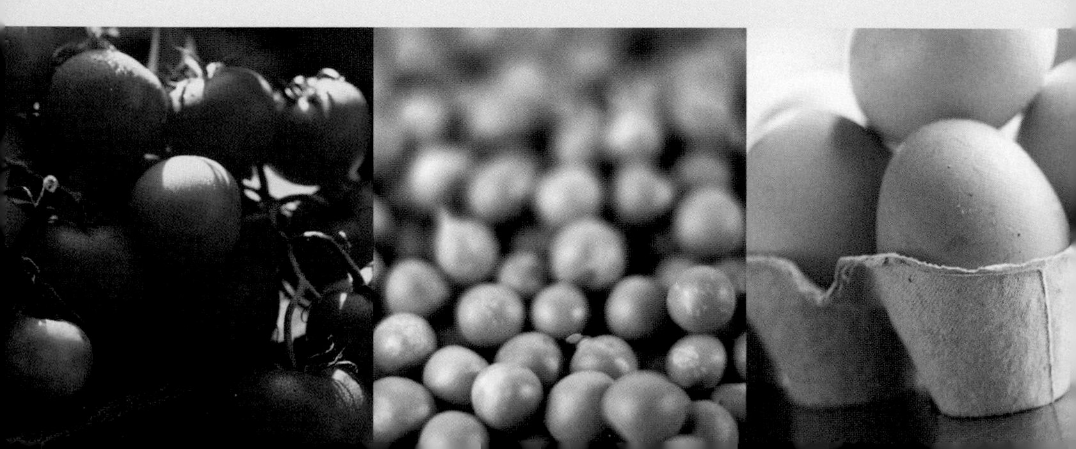

- Salmon
- Scallops
- Shrimp
- Steamed clams
- Turkey
- Veal
- Water-packed tuna

♥ FRESH VEGETABLES
(or canned, no additives)

- Asparagus
- Broccoli
- Brussels sprouts
- Cabbage
- Cauliflower
- Celery
- Chilies (green or red)
- Cucumber
- Eggplant
- Garlic
- Green beans
- Jalapeños
- Lettuce
- Olives
- Peppers (green, red, yellow)
- Pimentos
- Pumpkin
- Radishes
- Spinach
- Squash
- Sweet potatoes
- Tomatoes (all)
- Yams
- Zucchini

♥ MISCELLANEOUS
(no MSG or soy)

- Baking/cooking spices
- Baking powder
- Baking soda
- Bottled water
- Caffeine (2 servings a day or less than 100mg)
- Decaffeinated coffee
- Dry baking yeast
- Flour (unbleached, whole wheat)
- Garlic (cloves, powder)
- Honey
- Oil (canola, corn, olive)
- Onion (flakes, powder)
- Pepper (all)
- Purified tap water
- Salt
- Seafood cocktail sauce (no additives)
- Shortening (no soy)
- Spaghetti sauce (no additives)
- Tabasco sauce (no additives)
- Tomato juice (no additives)
- Tomato paste (no additives)
- Vanilla extract

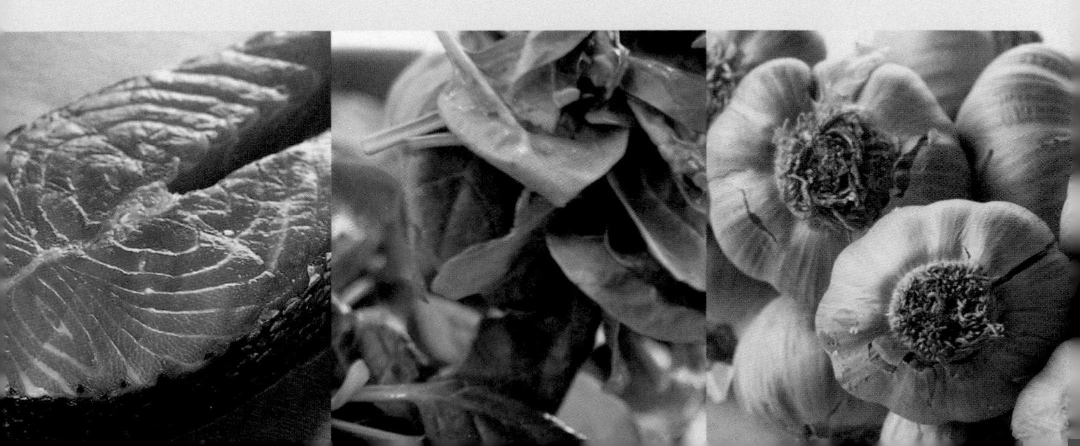

Q How can I eat enough protein if I am a vegetarian?

It may be diffuclt for those who depend upon vegetarian protein sources only, to get enough protein without using dairy products. You will need to use beans or legumes with the lowest tyramine content and avoid soy until you have control of your migraine attacks. Once you have control of your migraine you may return to using soy-based products. However, you will need to monitor your reaction closely for increase in migraine frequency. For those who are not vegetarians, soy and beans should be avoided until the migraine attacks are controlled for 8 months.

Q What do I do if everything I like to eat is on the trigger list?

There are many tasty foods on the migraine trigger list (see pp70–73). I struggle to stay away from many of them, especially when I have a stressful day. It is not simply the taste that makes the food so appetizing; it is also the sensation we experience after we eat them. It may be helpful to remind yourself that you are not giving up the pleasure of food forever, but simply until you have better migraine control. There are many delicious foods on the list of allowed foods (see pp91–93). It will be easier to change your eating habits if you concentrate on what you can eat and on your goal of headache-free days.

Q How do I avoid carbohydrates if my dinnertime is after 6.00pm?

It is important that you avoid food that has carbohydrates with a high glycemic index during the evening hours because these can cause hypoglycemia during your sleep and trigger a migraine attack. It will be helpful if you have protein and low carbohydrate vegetables easily available so you don't end up eating a bowl of cereal at night. You will need to review the allowed food list and make sure you have food available from the list designated with with the protein ♦ and free carbohydrate ♥ symbols.

Q How do I eat enough protein if my cholesterol is high or if I cannot eat dairy products?

You need to have protein with each serving of carbohydrate to avoid triggering a migraine attack. However, you do not have to eat excessive amounts of protein with excessive animal fat. You can use poultry and fish for most of your protein sources and limit the amount of red meat and egg yolks to avoid elevating your cholesterol levels. Those with complicated dietary needs will find a consultation with dietician helpful.

Q How much water do I need to drink and when?

It is crucial that you drink enough water to avoid dehydration and so avoid a migraine attack. You must drink at least 8 glasses of water a day. You may need to drink more water if you are very active or if you are in a hot, dry environment.

Q I do not cook, so how do I follow a migraine-friendly diet?

It is very important that you avoid pre-cooked packaged food since this type of food is likely to contain food additives that trigger a migraine attack. You may want to hire someone to cook for you or start by cooking simple, easy-to-prepare recipes.

Q How can I encourage my child to follow a migraine-friendly diet?

The child with migraine needs to understand that how and what he or she eats does have an effect on his or her headache frequency. Children need to have explained to them in terms they can understand how their eating habits can help them avoid a migraine attack. Start with simple changes, such as avoiding excessive carbohydrates, dehydration, and missing meals. Encourage the child to avoid food with additives. Lastly, restrict those food items that are more likely to trigger an attack, such as peanuts, chocolate, and citrus fruit.

Taking natural remedies

Q What vitamins, minerals, and supplements can help me control migraine attacks?

Several vitamins, minerals, and herbal supplements have been shown to be beneficial in treating migraine including magnesium, riboflavin (vitamin B_2), feverfew, coenzyme Q10, and butterbur root. However, all medicines, whether herbal, prescription, or non-prescription, have the potential for harm or benefit. You must discuss planned use of any product with your doctor. A natural product can still have "drug" effects and interact with other medications.

Q How does magnesium help with migraine?

As with prescription migraine medications, exactly how magnesium may help prevent a migraine is not well understood. Like the anticonvulsants prescribed for migraine, magnesium inhibits the spread of electrical activity across the brain. Some scientists think that migraine might be due to low magnesium levels. Doctors have found that 360–600mg of chelated (slow-release) oral magnesium oxide may help in migraine prevention; however, diarrhea may interfere with its uptake. Always check with your doctor before starting any supplements.

Q Does vitamin B_2 (riboflavin) help to prevent migraine?

One theory of migraine holds it to be a problem with mitochondria (the energy-producing part of a cell). Vitamin B_2 plays an important role in energy production by mitochondria; high doses of the vitamin might correct problems with this process and prevent migraine. Research has shown 25–400mg daily may help reduce migraine attacks. However, excessive use of B-complex vitamins to achieve the right dose of vitamin B_2 may be dangerous.

Q What is coenzyme Q10?

Coenzyme Q10 (CoQ10), like vitamin B_2, plays a role in energy production by mitochondria in cells. Research has suggested that CoQ10 may be helpful in preventing migraine attacks. The side effects reported during the studies included nausea, loss of appetite, indigestion, and diarrhea. Ask your doctor about CoQ10 before you start taking this supplement for migraine.

Q Some people have told me to take feverfew for my migraine. How can it help?

The leaves of the herb feverfew (*Tanacetum parthenium*) when dried and taken as a medicine, have an anti-inflammatory effect and work in a way similar to aspirin and other nonsteroidal anti-inflammatory drugs (NSAIDs), such as ibuprofen or naproxen. Feverfew may help in migraine by reducing constriction of blood vessels in the brain. Research has shown mixed results: some studies suggest it helps prevent attacks, while others disagree. Possible side effects include stomach upset and mouth ulcers and a "post-feverfew syndrome" of joint aches has been described, but it is unclear exactly what this is. Do not start feverfew without consulting your doctor. It is especially important not to mix it with NSAIDs since they cause the same side effects.

Q Can I take butterbur root to prevent migraine attacks?

The root of butterbur (*Petasites hybridus*), a shrub, is used in traditional remedies. Studies have shown that butterbur root is somewhat helpful in preventing migraine. It may work by blocking the inflammation process. However, the stem and leaves of the plant can cause cancer, liver disease, bleeding problems, and lung damage. For this reason, it is important to buy butterbur root only from a reputable source that has high safety standards. Again, talk to your doctor before using it.

Managing your stress

Q How can avoiding emotional stress help me prevent migraine attacks?

Reducing emotional stress is an important part of a comprehensive treatment program for treating migraine. Emotional stress causes increased levels of epinephrine, which speeds up brain activity, and is balanced by serotonin, which quiets brain activity. In people with migraine, serotonin activity is abnormal and brain cells become overexcited due to the effect of epinephrine. Think of each stressful situation as using your serotonin; you don't have enough to waste.

Q What role does serotonin play in my emotions?

Serotonin, a natural brain chemical, balances the activity of epinephrine, which is released during the stress response. Serotonin is the major neurotransmitter responsible for normal function of the limbic system, the part of the brain that creates our emotions. Without the right serotonin levels, the brain cannot function normally. Serotonin raises your mood, motivates you, and enables you to deal with problems. Without it, you may feel depressed, anxious, uninterested in life, and unable to concentrate.

Q How do I go about reducing the emotional stress in my life?

Reducing emotional stress is important both for the treatment of migraine and for your general health and well-being. To get started on a stress-reduction program, it is important to focus on 2 equally important approaches: stress prevention and stress management. Eliminating all stress in your life is an impossible goal since life is inherently stressful. You cannot predict every possible stressful situation, but maintaining a healthy lifestyle can prepare you to deal with unexpected stressors.

Q What is the difference between stress prevention and stress management?

Stress prevention is about establishing a biological, psychological, and spiritual program that helps you gain an optimal level of well-being that can prepare you to deal with future stressful situations when they occur. Stress management is your tool to help you solve a problem or deal with current emotional stress.

Q How do I get started with stress prevention and stress management?

The first step is to understand the connection between your biological response to stress (such as migraine) and the emotional situations. The biological response, called the stress, or "fight-or-flight," response causes an increase in epinephrine levels. If the level of epinephrine in your body stays raised for a period of time, it can cause harm to the body. Migraine is just one of many diseases that are adversely affected by stress. By maintaining good health with a healthy diet and regular exercise, you can prepare your body for this type of biological response. The next step is to learn more about how your emotions and behavior respond to stress and how, at times, they might add more to stress.

Q How do I learn more about my emotional and behavioral health?

There are many experts who can help you learn how to deal with emotional and behavioral issues. We all need to be aware of our emotional and psychological health; no one is born with an instruction manual on this. Understanding how we can change the way we think and behave can reduce the epinephrine levels and increase the serotonin levels in the brain. You may wish to seek professional help in the form of a counselor or therapist, and there are also many self-help books available. Ask your doctor if you are not sure where to get the best advice.

Myth "Frequent headaches, are a sign that you must be unhappy or stressed out"

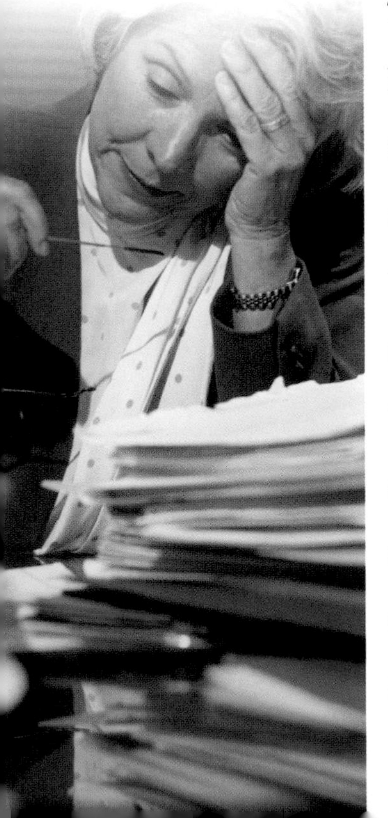

Truth Too many people have seen well-meaning healthcare professionals for their headaches, only to be told, on the basis of a normal brain scan, that "nothing is wrong; you only have migraine." The migraine sufferer is treated as though he or she is neurotic and needs to handle stress better. The truth is that migraine can be made worse by stress, but it is not caused by stress. Dismissing migraine headaches as a product of stress alone can cause sufferers to neglect the underlying triggers that cause their condition.

Q How can I prevent stress as a part of migraine treatment?

A comprehensive migraine treatment program must include a routine for relaxation and stress management. For best results, make this a daily routine. Giving yourself at least 30 minutes a day for a relaxation routine will help quiet your thoughts and reduce anxiety and epinephrine levels. Choose whatever works best for you: biofeedback, meditation, listening to music, reading, and so on. The important thing is to keep your concerns and the world outside at a distance for a while.

Q What if I am too busy to spend time on a relaxation program?

If that is your situation, it should give you a clue to why you are suffering from frequent migraine attacks. The most common reason for frequent migraine attacks from stress is an overcommitted schedule. People who are perfectionists or have problems delegating are often sufferers. There is also a tendency to try and make up for the lost time caused by attacks by overworking afterwards. Take a look at your schedule and reduce some of your commitments. It is important that you take care of yourself. A balanced life is the key; if stress in your life is generating too much epinephrine, it will adversely affect your migraine control.

Q How do I keep from feeling guilty for taking time for myself?

It is not uncommon for those with migraine to feel guilty for taking time off for exercise and relaxation because they think they have lost too much time to their migraine attacks already. However, you are actually making a time investment. When you take the time for stress management and exercise to prevent migraine attacks, you save the time you would otherwise have lost to a migraine attack. In addition, your stress management and exercise routine will boost your productivity so that you require less time to do the things you need to do.

Q How does being too busy trigger migraine attacks?

Migraine attacks can be triggered by anything that increases epinephrine release by brain cells, which are then overstimulated and require extra serotonin to calm down. Migraine is a "low-serotonin" disease; you cannot waste serotonin on hectic days and poor time management. You need to simplify your life to keep your epinephrine levels down and help you stop wasting serotonin.

Q How do I know what I need to do for stress management?

Determine the areas of your life that are causing you stress and try to resolve the problems you have identified. There may be areas of your life that cannot be "solved" and require you to accept the situation and unload resentment. You may need the help of a counselor or cognitive-behavioral therapy (CBT). Try to focus on the things that are most important and learn to let things go.

FIRST STEPS IN REDUCING STRESS

To start reducing stress in your life, you first need to identify stressful areas. Using the list of potential stress areas given below, write down all the issues that are causing you concern, anxiety, or fear. You can then make an effort to address each of these areas with the appropriate person or method. The important thing to remember is that nothing changes overnight, and that there will always be new challenges ahead.

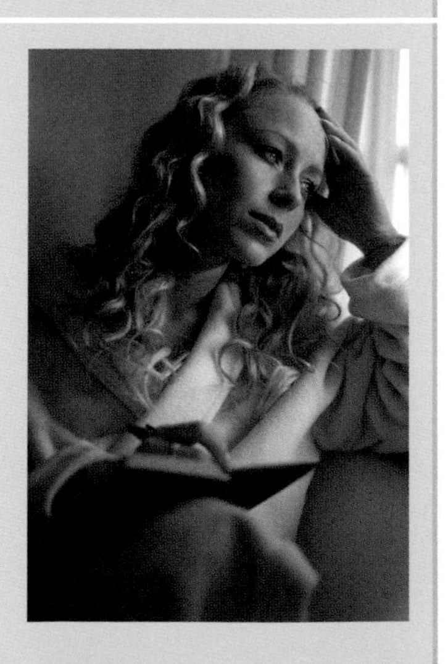

Potential Stress Areas:

• Work/school • Relationship issues • Financial
• Health • Community/national • Others

Physical activity

Q How can physical activity and exercise help me with my migraine treatment?

Regular physical activity and exercise give you what is called a "runner's high." This sensation of euphoria (elevated mood) is related to the release of brain chemicals called endorphins, which are natural painkillers. Regular exercise may also increase the levels of serotonin, although this area has not been well studied. It is known that regular exercise helps serotonin-related illnesses including depression, anxiety disorders, and migraine.

Q How do I go about adding a regular exercise program to my migraine treatment?

If you suffer from frequent migraine attacks, the idea of starting an exercise program may seem overwhelming. In addition, if you are in poor physical shape, intense exercise may trigger an attack. Frequently, people with severe migraine have not exercised in a long time, so it is important to start with an easy program. The important thing is to get started and do some physical activity every day.

Q What kind of exercise should I do?

Walking is a very effective exercise. Start with short walks and build up to 30–40 minutes a day. Avoid hypoglycemia (low blood sugar) and dehydration before and during exercise. A walking program for at least 6 months should significantly reduce the frequency of your migraine attacks.

Q How I can I stay committed to my exercise program?

Keeping a migraine diary (see p84) will help you recognize and keep track of improvement and will keep you motivated. You need to give exercise and treatment time to work. In time, your symptom-free life will more than reinforce your commitment to exercise.

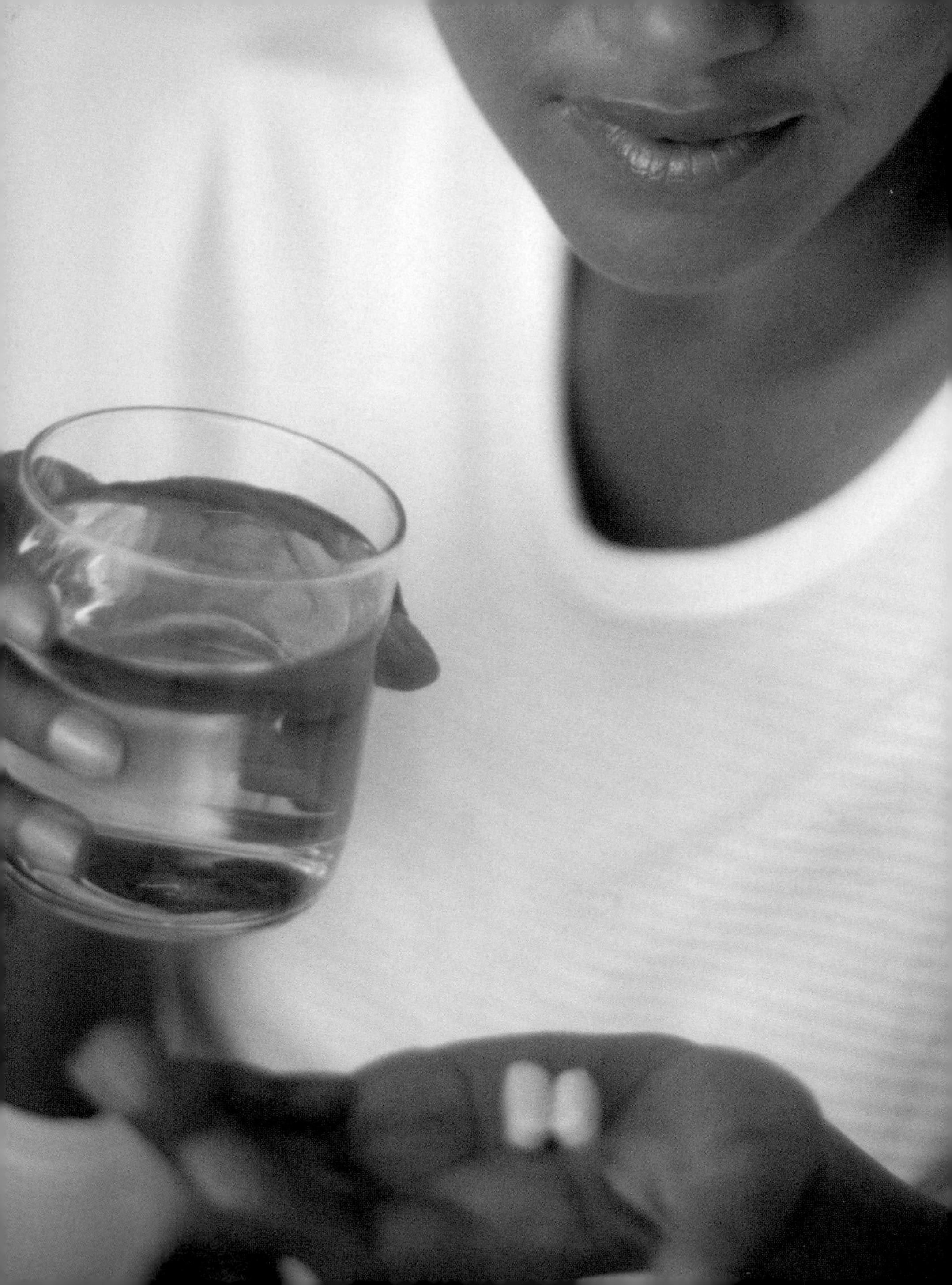

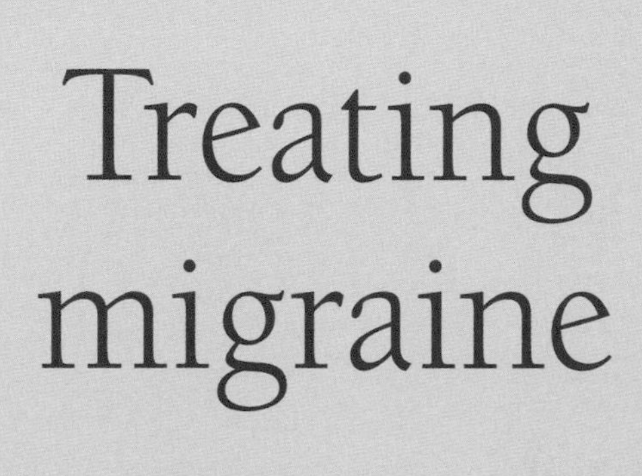

Treating migraine

The pain and suffering caused by a migraine attack is motivation enough for stopping it as soon as possible. However, taking steps to combat the symptoms and, more importantly, aborting an attack quickly and with the right fast-acting medication is crucial for treatment success.

The importance of timing

Q What should I do to stop a migraine attack?

The first thing you must do is take the attack seriously and treat it immediately. You will need to use a combination of approaches to abort (stop) an attack. An effective plan for aborting a migraine attack is to stop doing whatever you are doing and rest, take medication that can completely alleviate the headache and associated symptoms in less than 2 hours (see pp114–131), and avoid low blood sugar levels and dehydration. It is extremely important that all of this is done together and as soon as the attack starts.

Q I can usually ride out a headache. Do I need to treat a migraine attack?

Yes you do. Treating a migraine attack successfully is about time, not pain. As soon as you start to experience a migraine attack, you must stop the attack as quickly as possible; the longer you wait to treat the attack the more difficult it becomes to stop it. Your treatment for individual attacks is just as important as is the preventive treatment because the longer your migraine attack lasts, the more vulnerable you are to having another one.

Q Why does a migraine attack become more difficult to treat with time?

As a migraine attack progresses there are physiological changes (changes in body function) that can make the attack more difficult to treat. In the brain, the pain response system is disrupted, causing a cascade of pain responses that makes pain harder to control. In the digestive tract, there is a delay in emptying of the stomach, which affects the absorption of medications into the bloodstream (see p107).

Q How do changes in the brain during a migraine attack influence the effectiveness of medication?

Normally, the brain can reprogram its pain control system, much like a computer that has been loaded with "spam" or "pop ups." You can think of migraine attacks as "headache pop ups." Since migraine is a disruption of brain cell function, the longer the "migraine" program runs, the more "headache pop ups" happen to you. This process is called central sensitization (see p27). The development of central sensitization makes medication aimed at stopping an attack less effective; abortive medications are more likely to stop the headache completely when used before the cascade of pain responses of central sensitization starts. The only way to accomplish this goal and stop the headache is to take the medication early on in the attack and use the medication that works the best and fastest for you.

Q How do problems in digestive tract function affect medications aimed at stopping an attack?

Research studies have shown that during a migraine attack there is a delay in emptying of the stomach. The movement of stomach contents through the digestive tract is called gastric motility, and a delay in gastric motility is known as gastric stasis. The longer a migraine attack, the more severe the gastric stasis becomes. As a result, medications for treating migraine are not absorbed into the bloodstream as quickly and efficiently as they would be otherwise. For this reason, a migraine attack cannot be completely stopped if there is a delay in treatment.

Q Can gastric stasis affect medications other than those I take for migraine?

This is a very good question but one that has not been properly studied. If you are having frequent migraine attacks, which we know influences the absorption of migraine medication, then it is possible that any medication taken in pill form could be similarly affected.

Q Why can't I just wait for the headache to get bad enough before I take my medication?

To treat migraine effectively, you need to understand that it is a "time thing not a pain thing." Many people wait for the headache to get "bad enough" before they take their medication. Over the years I have heard every reason possible for not treating attacks when they start, from "it might go away" to "I am afraid I will run out of medicine" or "I will use too much medicine." The fact is that migraine will not magically go away and, furthermore, the longer you wait the more likely it is that you will have more attacks. Overusing an abortive medication is a reasonable concern, which is why migraine prevention is as important as the treatment. However, when you do have an attack, any delay in treatment allows progression of central sensitization, in which an increasing number of sensory nerves are recruited into the pain process, making the attack more difficult to treat. The longer you wait, the more vulnerable you will be to further attacks.

Q How do I deal with other people who think it is "just a headache" and do not understand why I must stop what I am doing and treat my migraine attack?

Dealing with those around who do not understand migraine can be very challenging. Do not take on this kind of challenge during a migraine attack—it wastes time and causes more stress. Take care of yourself and the migraine attack first and deal with people later. Many people who do not suffer from migraine do not understand that the illness is about more than just pain. Taking the time to educate the people in your life about your condition is very important, but you only need to educate them, not change their belief system. You do not have to make excuses for your illness. It is what it is. People must accommodate your illness just as they would any other chronic medical condition, such as asthma or diabetes.

Q What if I cannot leave work or stop whatever I am doing to treat a migraine attack?

If you address a migraine attack early on in the process with aggressive, effective treatment you will rarely need to stop what you are doing for long periods of time. There are very few jobs or projects during which you cannot stop for a few minutes to treat the attack. If your job is so important that you cannot stop to treat a migraine, then it is certainly too important to do with a migraine attack. Migraine is not simply a headache. The disruption in brain function during an attack affects your job performance. In addition, the longer you wait to treat a migraine attack the more attacks you will have and the more your job and life will be adversely affected.

Q Is it important for children to treat their migraine attacks early?

Yes, children and teenagers often delay treatment of their migraine attacks to the point where they become very ill. They are often reluctant or fearful of asking a teacher to excuse them from class to go see the school nurse. Parents may encourage this behavior because they are concerned about their child using medication. Yet very often, all that is needed early in the attack is rest, food, and water. If medication is needed to treat a migraine attack, delaying treatment will simply mean that more medication will be required. Children, like adults, can go on to develop chronic migraine (headaches on more than 15 days a month) so it is crucial that attacks be contained.

Q What if the migraine attack starts while I am sleeping?

Migraine attacks can happen during sleep and place you at risk of a very severe attack. When you wake from sleep with a migraine attack, it is crucial that you start treatment quickly. You may find the attack very difficult to treat. If it continues for 2 hours after treatment, it is very important that you treat it again even if it is "better."

Eating and drinking

Q Does it make a difference if I eat during a migraine attack?

Yes, it does make a difference. You do not have to eat or drink very much; the nausea and vomiting associated with a migraine attack may make it difficult. However, the longer you wait to eat or drink, the more nausea you will experience. Many people believe that eating or drinking will make the nausea worse. This is incorrect: your stomach is not causing the nausea; the nausea and vomiting are symptoms of the attack. The longer you go without eating, the more severe your hypoglycemia becomes and the worse the migraine attack and nausea.

Q What can I eat or drink when I have a migraine attack?

First, keep it simple. The last thing you will want to do is prepare food. It is important that you have some carbohydrate, protein, and water, but do not have the carbohydrate without protein. Many people will sip juice and eat crackers, only to fuel their migraine with a sugar buzz. It is easier to take small amounts frequently. You can try toast or crackers with mild cheese, turkey, or chicken. Drink at least 8 ounces of water an hour until the migraine attack stops. Increase water intake if you are vomiting.

Q What if I'm in a situation where I can't eat or drink something?

It is important that you keep your "headache snack" and water readily available along with your abortive medication. Treating a migraine attack immediately is as important as treating a low blood sugar episode is for someone with diabetes. If you are in a situation where you cannot have your "headache snack," proceed with your medication and water. It is important that you stop what you are doing for a while as soon as posssible and eat.

Relaxation

Q How important is rest or relaxation in the treatment of a migraine attack?

It may be tempting to take a pill and continue with the task at hand during an attack, but this may make things worse. A migraine attack is caused by excitation of brain cells and to reduce this excitation you must stop stimulating these cells. It doesn't take long to stop an attack if you act quickly. You must treat the migraine attack as soon as it starts and not wait for it to get worse.

Q How should I relax?

There are many relaxation techniques you can use to help abort a migraine attack (see pp112–113). The one you choose needs to fit your personality and belief system. You may want to learn formal relaxation methods such as meditation or biofeedback techniques. If you are a person of faith, you might use prayer. You may want to listen to music or audio books. It is important that you avoid visual stimuli so I would suggest that you do not read, watch television, or work on a computer. For some people a massage is helpful; for others the last thing they want is to be touched. Relaxation is a personal matter, so whatever works for you is the method to use.

Q How important is one's environment for relaxation during a migraine attack?

Reducing environmental stimuli during a migraine attack helps reduce brain excitation. Resting in a quiet, dark, scent-free place will help to stop a migraine attack. Even if you cannot find such a place, it is important to pause, treat the attack, and sit back with closed eyes for 5–15 minutes. If the attack continues for more than 2 hours, you will need to repeat your medications, stop activity completely, and rest.

Relaxation techniques

Relaxation is an important part of getting well. It helps break the vicious cycle of pain and stress, and brings various physiological benefits, such as decreased levels of epinephrine, sugar, and cholesterol in the blood, and improved lung function and metabolic rate. Many techniques have been developed to help with relaxation.

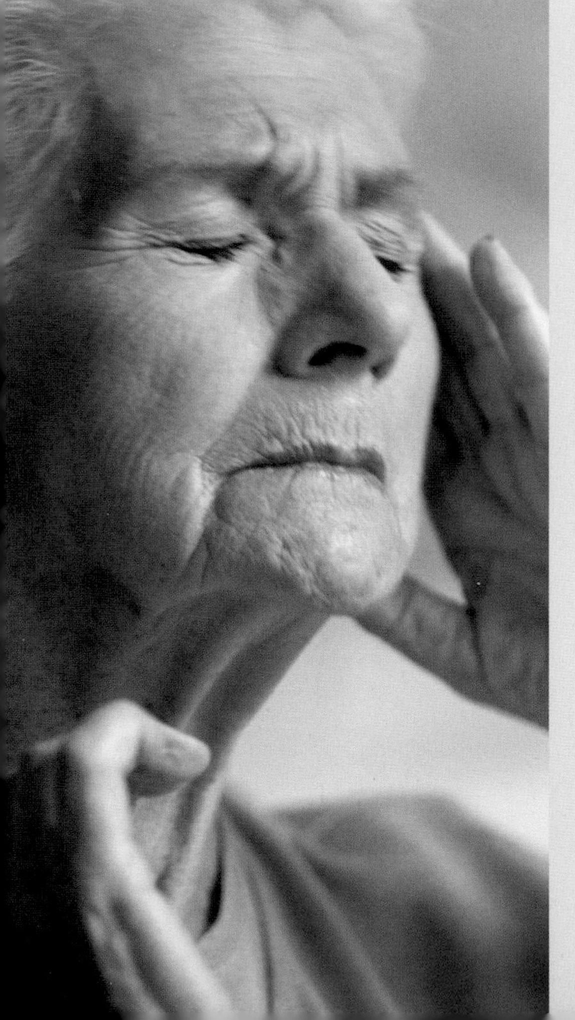

DEEP BREATHING

When a migraine attack starts, sit up straight but don't breathe forcefully. Instead, breathe in gently and let your chest expand fully.

Relax your neck and shoulders.

Put either hand on your stomach just above your navel and below your ribcage.

Breathe in slowly and deeply through your nose. As you do so, feel your hand and stomach gently rising up.

As soon as your lungs are full, breath out through your mouth slowly and steadily. At the same time, feel your hand and stomach gently falling.

Repeat this cycle of breathing in and out 4 or 5 times, then rest. Breathe normally in a relaxed way for a couple of minutes. If you feel you need to, repeat the sequence for 5 more minutes.

PROGRESSIVE RELAXATION

Sit quietly and close your eyes.

First relax the muscles in your toes and feet, then work your way up your legs to your stomach, hands, arms, shoulders, and finally your neck. Try to keep the muscles relaxed as you work your way up your body.

Take gentle breaths through your nose and focus on your breathing as you inhale and exhale.

Breathe normally for 10 minutes or so, focusing on your breathing for as long as you can. To help you keep distracting thoughts at bay, repeat a word such as "one" every time you breathe out.

When you've finished the exercise, sit quietly with your eyes closed. Continue to focus on your breathing if it helps you relax.

MUSCLE RELAXATION

Stop what you're doing and lie down in a quiet place. If you can't lie down, sit or stand quietly while you do the exercise.

If your breathing is shallow and quick, breathe deeply a few times.

Close your eyes and imagine a relaxing scene, such as sitting on a hillside, looking at a beautiful landscape.

Tighten the muscles in your shoulders, hold them tight for 5 seconds, and then relax. You should be able to feel the release of tension in the muscles and joints. You might get a sense that they are a little bit looser and you are lighter.

Repeat this tightening and relaxing sequence with as many muscle groups as you can—from your shoulders, arms, and stomach to your legs and toes.

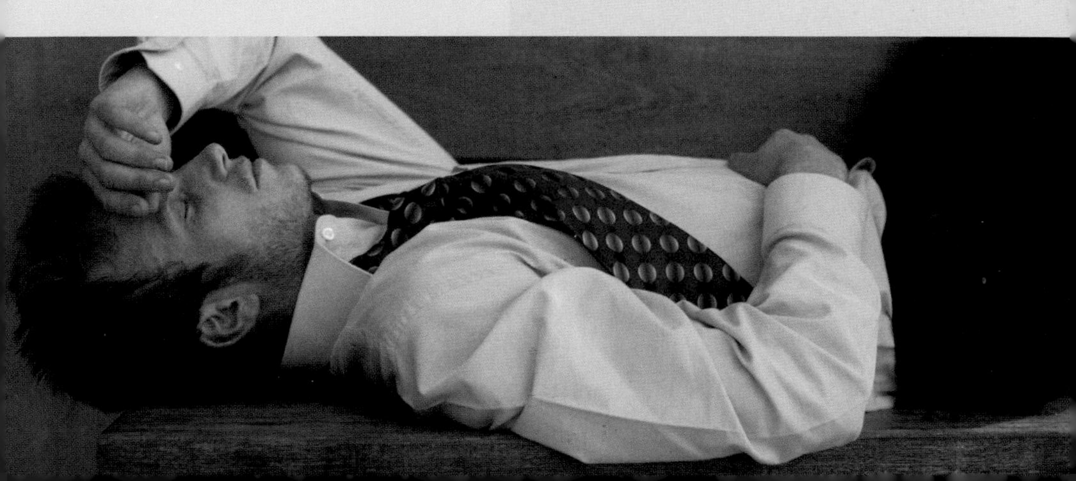

Treatment with medications

Q I understand the importance of aborting a migraine attack early but what do I use to treat it?

There are a couple of possible approaches to treating your migraine: you may use analgesics to ease or relieve your pain or you may use abortive medications to stop the migraine attack. You can buy analgesics, such as acetaminophen, and some abortive medications, such as ibuprofen and aspirin, over the counter without a prescription. Stronger, more powerful medications —both analgesics and abortive drugs—require a doctor's prescription. Before you decide to treat your headaches and migraine attacks yourself, it is important that you have the diagnosis of migraine confirmed by a doctor.

Q I have a headache every day that I treat with over-the-counter analgesics but only have a migraine attack 4 to 8 times a month. Do I have medication overuse headache?

You may very well. Medication overuse headache can potentially be caused by either analgesics or abortive migraine medication. However, you can only confirm the diagnosis by stopping the medication in question and waiting to see if the daily headache disappears. Medication overuse is the most important risk factor for developing chronic daily headache (more than 15 headache days a month) and accounts for around 80 percent of those suffering from chronic daily headache. The overuse of analgesics or abortive medications hinders the effectiveness of migraine preventive medications. The treatment of severe migraine complicated with long-standing medication overuse requires the expertise of a headache specialist or a doctor experienced in treating severe headache disorders. It is not enough simply to treat the symptoms of a migraine attack or to abort it—you must prevent frequent attacks.

MEDICATIONS USED TO TREAT A MIGRAINE ATTACK

The medications used to treat a migraine attack can be classified into 2 main groups: those that treat the pain are called nonspecific and those that abort the attack are called specific. Medications used to treat the pain of a migraine attack are classified as simple analgesics, combination analgesics, or opioid analgesics. Specific medications used to abort a migraine attack are nonsteroidal anti-inflammatory drugs (NSAIDs), triptans, and ergotamine-related medications. Note that aspirin is classified both as an NSAID and an analgesic. Medications that are used to treat nausea and vomiting (antiemetics) or cause relaxation (sedatives) are referred to as adjunctive therapies.

NONSPECIFIC MEDICATIONS (PAIN RELIEF)	
Simple analgesics: Acetaminophen	Available over the counter
Combination analgesics: Aspirin or acetaminophen combined with other drugs	Many available over the counter
Opioid analgesics	Prescription only

SPECIFIC MEDICATIONS (ABORTIVE THERAPY)	
Nonsteroidal anti-inflammatory drugs (NSAIDs), including aspirin	Some available over the counter; most are prescription only
Triptans	Prescription only
Ergotamine-related medications	Prescription only

ADJUNCTIVE THERAPIES	
Antiemetics	Prescription only
Sedatives	Prescription only

Q I take a medication for headache 4 to 5 times per week, but I do not think I have migraine. How can I know for sure?

You will need to stop taking your frequent medication in order to establish whether you have migraine or another headache disorder. You should also consult a doctor to make sure you do not have another medical disorder contributing to your frequent headaches. If you have migraine and you have stopped overusing abortive medications, you will find that you then start to have more typical migraine attacks. The overuse of abortive medication changes the symptoms of migraine and makes headaches appear as though they are tension or sinus-related headaches or even "daily" migraine.

Q What do people with migraine want their headache medication to do?

Studies have shown that people with migraine want the same thing their doctors do when it comes to headache relief or abortive medications: they want their medication to be effective. It needs to provide rapid and complete relief from the migraine attack and there should be no recurrence of the attack. People with migraine want the medication to be in tablet or capsule form and obviously prefer medications with no side effects.They do not want to have to be concerned about an attack preventing them from participating in work, social, or family activities.

Q How do I know whether I need a prescription medication or an over-the-counter drug?

You can determine your need for a prescription medication over one you can purchase over the counter by the effectiveness of the medication. If the over-the-counter medication completely aborts the migraine attack in less than 2 hours, then you do not need a prescription medication. However, if your attacks last longer than 2 hours, you do need to use a prescription migraine medication. This approach is called stratified care.

Q Why do I need my abortive medication to relieve my headache within 2 hours?

You will need to abort the migraine attack as quickly as possible, since the longer you have a headache, the more the attack progresses. When you stop the headache, you treat the disease and help prevent the next attack. Severe migraine may require prescription medication to ensure that the attacks are stopped soon.

EFFECTIVE TREATMENT

Headache-free results are more easily achieved when the attack is treated before central sensitization (see p27) occurs. You will receive the greatest benefit from your migraine medication if you intervene early in the attack and use a fast-acting, effective medication that brings lasting relief. The medication should also be safe and ideally, should have no side effects. It may take time to find the right medication or the combination of medications needed to effectively treat your migraine attacks. Many of your migraine attacks may be mild enough to treat with over-the-counter medications such as acetaminophen, ibuprofen, or aspirin. However, more severe attacks will require prescription medication. Using effective abortive therapy (NSAIDs, triptans, or ergotamine-related medication) will reduce your need for excessive medication.

FAST RELIEF

Medication must start to work quickly

Medication should provide headache-free response within 2 hours

LASTING RELIEF

There should be low recurrence rates (headache does not return next day)

It should provide sustained headache-free response (headache does not return within 24 hours)

It should give consistent headache-free response (medication works for all attacks)

SAFETY AND TOLERABILITY

It should be safe for you to use

It should cause no or little sedation, or difficulty concentrating

There should be minimal or transient side effects

Over-the-counter pain relief

Q What medications can I purchase without a prescription to relieve the pain of a migraine attack?

Several over-the-counter medications called analgesics can relieve the pain of the headache during a migraine attack. Many analgesics consist of acetaminophen alone and are known as simple analgesics. Others may be a combination of aspirin or acetaminophen with caffeine, decongestants, and/or antihistamines. These combination analgesics are marketed for migraine, tension headache, or sinus headache. In countries outside the US, you can buy analgesics with a mix of acetaminophen and codeine.

Q What do I need to know about the use of analgesics for my migraine attacks?

Analgesics are nonspecific medications and should only be used for the treatment of a migraine attack when more specific medications cannot be used. If you do use analgesics to relieve the pain of a migraine attack, you must not use them more than once a week or you might develop medication overuse headache (see p78).

Q Why do companies market so many over-the-counter drugs for different types of headache?

Headache is a very common ailment so it has a large consumer market. There are many heavily advertised brand-name products for those suffering from different types of headache. People who have headaches with neck tightness are sold a tension headache pill. If they have headaches over the forehead associated with congestion, they are sold a sinus headache pill. These brand-name products can be expensive and often contain compounds (such as caffeine, decongestants, or antihistamines) not needed to treat a migraine headache. It is important that you have a correct diagnosis for your headache so that you can avoid unnecessary medication and expense.

Q Is it enough just to stop the pain of an attack?

As discussed earlier, abortive therapy is very important, so medication used to treat an attack must be effective. It is not enough to decrease the pain. You must completely stop the attack. Nonspecific medications simply treat the symptoms rather than the underlying cause and increase vulnerability to medication overuse headache (see p78).

NONSPECIFIC OVER-THE-COUNTER TREATMENT

To relieve the pain of a migraine attack you can use acetaminophen alone (a simple analgesic) or acetaminophen combined with other drugs (a combination analgesic).

SIMPLE ANALGESICS: Acetaminophen is an over-the-counter analgesic for pain relief. When you can't use aspirin or other NSAIDs due to illnesses or pregnancy, acetaminophen alone, or in a combination analgesic, can treat migraine pain. The use of prescription migraine abortive therapy (see p126) is needed if you use analgesics more than 3 times a month.

TYPICAL DOSAGE:

- Acetaminophen 650mg

COMBINATION ANALGESICS: Some combination analgesics contain caffeine, aspirin, and/or a mild opioid and are marketed for tension headache. Others contain diphenhydramine (an antihistamine) or decongestants and are marketed for sinus headache.

The combination analgesics with a mild opioid such as codeine are not available over the counter in the US. By combining the medications each drug enhances the effect of the others, providing better pain relief. The most popular over-the-counter combination analgesics in the US are those that contain acetaminophen, caffeine, and aspirin. However, this type of drug is one of the leading causes of medication overuse headache.

TYPICAL DOSAGE:

- Aspirin 325mg, caffeine 40mg, and acetaminophen 325mg
- Acetaminophen 325mg, caffeine 40mg
- Acetaminophen 325mg and diphenhydramine (an antihistamine) 25mg
- Acetaminophen 325mg and different products containing decongestants

Over-the-counter abortive therapy

Q What are the most effective over-the-counter medications to stop a migraine attack?

Aspirin and other nonsteroidal anti-inflammatory drugs (NSAIDs), such as ibuprofen and naproxen, are particularly helpful once central sensitization has started. It is important to avoid overusing these medications since you could develop gastrointestinal or kidney problems.

Q How do aspirin and the other NSAIDs work to treat a migraine attack?

Aspirin and the other NSAIDs are considered a specific treatment because they treat the process of the migraine attack, not simply the pain of the headache. It is thought that their anti-inflammatory properties work at the brain cell level or block chemical release at nerve endings, preventing the inflammation and dilation of blood vessels.

Q How do I know if I am taking too much aspirin or other NSAIDs for my migraine attacks?

If you are using aspirin or another NSAID more than twice a week for your attacks, then you are taking too much. Migraine attacks aborted with any kind of therapy should not occur more than twice a week or you can progress to chronic daily headache. It is not enough to use abortive therapy for migraine; you must have preventive care too.

Q Can my child take an NSAID or aspirin for a migraine attack?

Aspirin is not recommended for those under 18 because of the potential for Reye syndrome, and acetaminophen might cause medication overuse headache. However, children and teenagers may use other NSAIDs for migraine attacks. Consult your doctor about the proper dose for your child.

SPECIFIC OVER-THE-COUNTER TREATMENT

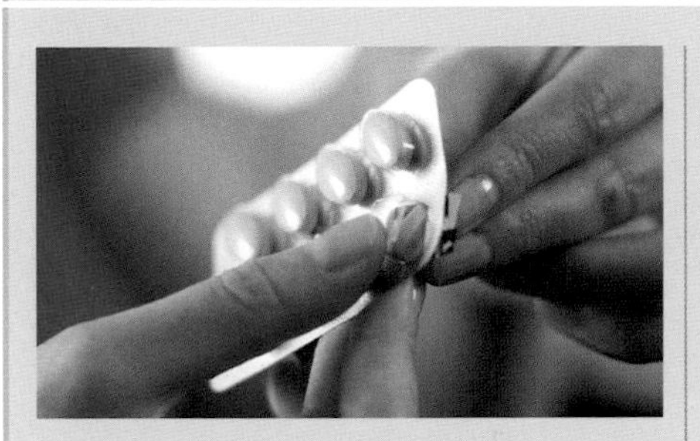

The most effective over-the-counter medications for aborting a migraine attack are aspirin, ibuprofen, and naproxen sodium. These nonsteroidal anti-inflammatory drugs (NSAIDs) block the chemical reaction in the body that produces inflammation. Originally used to treat the inflammation and pain of arthritis, these medications have now been found to be very helpful in treating many illnesses, including migraine attacks. These medications do not simply treat the pain of a migraine attack but stop the process of the attack.

If the migraine is not successfully aborted within 2 hours or less using aspirin or another NSAID, then these medications need to be combined with specific migraine abortive therapy (either triptans or dihydroergtamine) which is only available on prescription (see pp126–129 for more details).

OVER-THE-COUNTER NSAIDS

- Aspirin 1,000mg
- Ibuprofen 600–800mg
- Naproxen sodium 440–660mg (available over-the-counter in the US but may require a prescription in some other countries)

SAFE USE OF NSAIDS

To avoid gastrointestinal upset, NSAIDs should be taken with food and a large glass of water.

The overuse of NSAIDs can cause stomach problems and should be avoided if you have medical problems associated with gastrointestinal bleeding or ulcers, or if you are taking medications that interact with NSAIDs (ask you doctor if you are not sure).

The NSAIDs, apart from aspirin, can complicate high blood pressure and heart disease; do not use these drugs without consulting your doctor.

As with all over-the-counter medications, if you have other chronic medical conditions you should never self-medicate with anything before consulting your doctor.

When to see your doctor

Q I've tried over-the-counter medications to treat my migraine attacks but they don't seem to be working. Is it time to see my doctor?

Over-the-counter medications can be considered effective for abortive migraine therapy when they completely stop an attack in 2 hours or less. If you have migraine attacks that are not aborted in 2 hours, or if an attack recurs, you need to see your doctor to find out what the problem is. He or she may prescribe more potent medication for your abortive therapy. Nearly all of your migraine attacks must be limited to 2 hours or less and occur no more than twice a week or you are at risk of chronic daily headache.

Q How important is it that I choose the "right" doctor for my migraine treatment?

Using prescription medication for your attacks requires that you see a doctor who knows how to treat people with migraine. Although medical schools and hospitals are trying to better educate students about migraine, not all doctors know as much about migraine as they need to. All too often people with headaches are evaluated for a "real disease" causing their headaches, then simply given a pain pill when tests show no evidence of disease. You may need to research the appropriate treatment program. For helpful information about websites and headache organizations see p184.

Q Why do people wait so long before they go to a doctor about their migraine?

Many migraine sufferers are unaware of the advancements in migraine treatment and believe that nothing can be done about their headaches. Some believe their headaches are a "normal" part of their life, while others put off seeing a doctor until attacks become so frequent and severe they are forced to seek medical help. In fact, it is much better to seek help early, before problems become chronic.

Q Are there different medical approaches to treating a migraine attack?

When your doctor prescribes a treatment plan for your migraine attack, he or she can use either of a couple of possible approaches: stratified care (the use of different medications depending on the severity of your attacks) or step care (which is the use of the same medications everytime).

Q How does stratified care of a migraine attack work?

Stratified care is a method of treating a migraine attack based upon the severity of the attack and the level of disability it causes. For example, if the migraine attack starts out slowly with a mild headache during the day, then you could abort it with a simple analgesic. But, if you were to wake in the middle of the night suffering from a full-blown migraine with severe headache and vomiting, you might need a self-injectable migraine medication and a rectal suppository for vomiting. It is important to use the method that is the most effective for aborting the attack as soon as possible. It is not enough to feel better; you must stop the attack otherwise your migraine could get worse.

Q What is step care of a migraine attack?

When step care is used to treat a migraine attack, the same therapy is used no matter how the attack starts. If the therapy does not work it is changed. This approach is less effective than stratified care because it may lead to the prolonged use of ineffective medication or poorly tolerated drugs. Studies have shown that stratified care provides a better treatment response than step care. If the therapy you are using does not abort the headache completely in less than 2 hours or if your migraine attack recurs, you must change your abortive approach. The ineffective treatment of migraine attacks can cause progression of migraine and the development of chronic daily headache.

Myth "It is OK to use over-the-counter medications as often as I want"

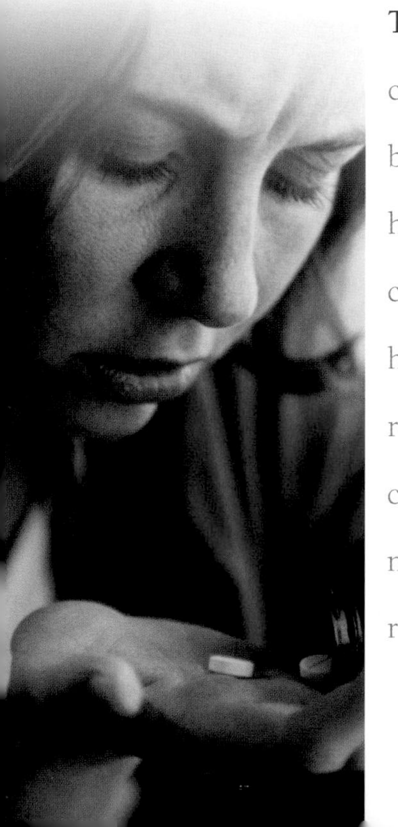

Truth Many people who take over-the-counter medications for what they believe to be tension (stress-related) headache or sinus headache have mild to moderate headaches caused by migraine. They may feel it is not harmful as long as they do not exceed the recommended dosage. If you use over-the-counter tension or sinus headache medications more than a couple of days a week, you are at risk of medication overuse headache.

Prescription pain relief

Q When is it appropriate to use prescription analgesics for migraine attacks?

Analgesics, both simple and combination, must be avoided, unless no other medications are available. During pregnancy and for people who cannot take triptans, ergotamine-related medications, or NSAIDs, the use of prescription analgesics may be the only option. If analgesics are used, they must be limited to no more than twice a month. They should never be the first choice for attacks simply because they are cheap as overuse can lead to medication overuse headaches.

PRESCRIBED ANALGESICS

Medications that are prescribed to combat the pain of migraine may be combination analgesics or an opioid analgesic on its own. The combination analgesics consist of acetaminophen and/or aspirin together with one or more of the following: caffeine, codeine, or sedatives (butalbital, isometheptene, or dichloralaphenazone).

Prescribed analgesics are generally much stronger than their over-the-counter equivalents. They should be taken carefully and never excessively because if they are overused they can cause more headaches and also place you at significant risk of addiction.

OPIOIDS

- Hydrocodone 5mg
- Codeine 30–60mg

COMBINATION ANALGESICS

- Acetaminophen 325mg with caffeine 40mg and codeine 30mg
- Aspirin 325mg or acetaminophen 325mg with caffeine 40mg plus butalbital 50mg with or without codeine 30mg
- Acetaminophen 325mg, isometheptene 65mg, and dichloralaphenazone 100mg

Prescription abortive therapy

Q Which prescription medications are used to stop a migraine attack?

Prescription medications used to abort migraine attacks include NSAIDs, triptans, ergotamine, and dihydroergotamine. These medications may be used alone, in combination with each other, or with adjunctive therapy, depending upon the attack. The headache and associated symptoms of a migraine attack vary; therefore your abortive therapy regimen also needs to be flexible.

Q How will I know which medication to use?

Several prescription medications can be used for abortive migraine treatment. Your doctor must tailor your abortive therapy to your attacks. This may take time and means trying various medications until you find a medication that completely aborts your attacks in 2 hours or less.

Q How will I know when to use my abortive therapy?

You need to use your abortive medication as soon as a migraine attack starts. During a migraine attack, you develop gastric stasis (delayed emptying of the stomach), which decreases absorption of medications. Abortive medication must be absorbed into the bloodstream quickly for it to stop a migraine attack.

Q How often can I take medications for a migraine attack?

You should not overuse abortive therapy. Ideally, you should not have to use your abortive therapy more than 1 day a week. If you are experiencing more than 1 attack a week then you need preventive medication, or a medication change if you are using preventive therapy.

Q How can I be more confident about my migraine attack treatment?

An effective abortive therapy is the key. It secures you in the knowledge that if and when you have a migraine attack, you can control it, instead of getting stressed and triggering another attack. As time passes, you will become more confident in your abortive therapy.

PRESCRIBED NSAIDS

Most NSAIDs, except aspirin, ibuprofen, and naproxen sodium, require a prescription. If the migraine is not aborted in 2 hours or less with aspirin or other NSAIDs, then these medications need to be combined with another migraine abortive therapy, using either triptans (see p126) or dihydroergotamine (see p129).

NSAID	FORM	DOSAGE
Tolfenamic acid	pill	1,000mg
Pirprofen	pill	200mg
Indometacin	suppository	75–100mg
Ketoprofen	suppository	100mg
Diclofenac	suppository	75mg
Ketorolac	injection	60mg

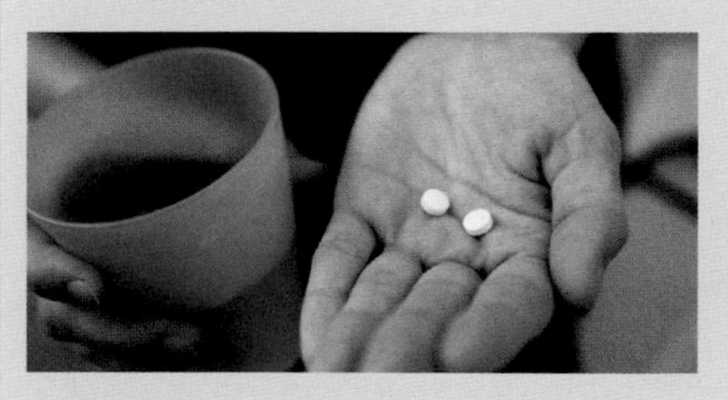

SAFE USE OF NSAIDS

NSAIDs in pill form should be taken with food and water to avoid gastrointestinal upset.

The overuse of NSAIDs can cause stomach problems and should be avoided if you have medical problems associated with gastro-intestinal bleeding or ulcers, and/or are taking medications that interact with NSAIDs.

NSAIDs can complicate high blood pressure and heart disease; make sure your doctor knows if you have one of these medical conditions.

Q What are triptans?

The triptans are a group of medications that abort the migraine process and stop the headache of a migraine attack. Their effectiveness is time-dependent; if triptans are used too late in an attack they do not work well. The addition of triptans to your abortive treatment can help with the final step in "switching off" the migraine attack.

Q How do triptans work?

The triptans "switch off" a migraine attack. A migraine attack occurs because the "calming" brain chemical serotonin does not function properly, resulting in the overactivity of brain cells and nerves. The triptans work like serotonin, attaching themselves to serotonin receptors and "switching off" the brain cells and nerves that are excited during a migraine attack.

Q Are there different types of triptan?

There are several different triptans: almotriptan, eletriptan, frovatriptan, naratriptan, rizatriptan, sumatriptan, and zolmitriptan. Each can be very effective, although they vary in effectiveness among different people: what works for one person may be less helpful for another. Your doctor will supervise you while you try each one to determine which triptan is best for your migraine attack and has the least side effects.

Q Can medications combine a triptan and an NSAID together?

Yes. There is a new combination pill containing sumatriptan and naproxen that is pending approval from the Food & Drug Administration (FDA). It makes use of technology that allows the different medications to be absorbed in a timely fashion. The triptan is absorbed quickly to allow it to stop the migraine. The NSAID has been changed to be absorbed quickly but stay longer in the blood, allowing the pill to better abort the attack.

Q What are the potential side effects of triptans?

The common side effects caused by the use of triptans are tingling, warmth, dizziness, flushing, chest discomfort, and sensations of pressure. These side effects vary from one person to another. One of the triptans may cause you to experience side effects while another does not. The side effects do not cause harm and usually last only a few minutes. People with medication overuse headache may experience more intense side effects.

Q What are the safety precautions for the use of triptans?

Triptans can cause coronary vasospasm (spasm of arteries in the heart), and therefore should not be given to people with coronary artery disease or who have had a heart attack or to people with symptoms or findings that indicate significant underlying cardiovascular disease. The triptans can raise blood pressure so they should not be given to people with uncontrolled hypertension. Hemiplegic and basilar migraine (see chart, pp16–19) should not be treated with triptans, and triptans should not be used during pregnancy. You need to avoid using different triptans, or a triptan and an ergotamine-related medication, on the same day.

Q How are ergotamine and dihydroergotamine used to treat migraine attacks?

Medications containing ergotamine are now rarely used because of the development of triptans. However, dihydroergotamine can be especially effective for severe migraine and migraine of long duration, such as menstrual migraine. Dihydroergotamine is available in the form of a nasal spray and an injectable formulation. The dose for the nasal spray is 5mg and the dose for the injectable formulation is 0.5–1mg. Ergotamine causes significant nausea and has more potential for causing artery spasm than does dihydroergotamine.

Prescription adjunctive therapy

Q What is an adjunctive medication?

When a medication is used to treat a symptom of the condition, but not for treatment of the condition itself, it is called an adjunctive medication. In the treatment of migraine attacks, adjunctive medications can be used to treat nausea and vomiting or to cause sedation.

Q Can adjunctive medications help with a migraine attack?

Yes. Some adjunctive medications can help abort a migraine attack because they act as sedatives (make you sleepy). Sleep can abort a migraine attack. Many anti-nausea medications cause sedation in addition to stopping nausea and vomiting and so can also help with the attack.

Q How do antiemetics help during migraine attacks?

During an attack, nausea and vomiting can prevent you from eating or cause dehydration, which may make the attack last longer. Antiemetics (antinausea medications) will help you keep down food and liquids and can relieve the discomfort of nausea.

Q How are sedatives used to treat migraine?

Sedatives are frequently prescribed for migraine attacks. However, they should be avoided because they can cause medication overuse headache. In some cases, sedation can be crucial. If a severe attack is not aborted within 2 hours with your usual medication, you need to repeat your initial medication and add something to make you sleepy. In this case, taking an antinausea medication that causes sedation will help you sleep and is better than taking a sedative.

Q Is there a medication I can use for nausea that does not cause sedation?

Yes, you can use metoclopramide. This prescription medication does not cause sedation and can help with the absorption of your abortive migraine medications. You can take it with your abortive medications.

DRUGS TO TREAT NAUSEA AND VOMITING

The most effective medication for the nausea and vomiting of a migraine attack is one that can alleviate the symptoms as quickly as possible. It is very important that these symptoms are controlled as soon as possible so you can drink water and eat. If you are unable to avoid hypoglycemia and dehydration, the migraine attack will worsen. Effective medication for nausea and vomiting must be available at all times. You will need to discuss the use of these medications with your doctor.

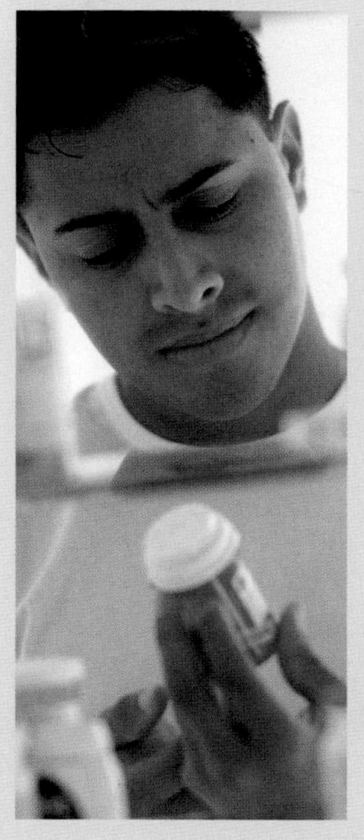

ANTIEMETIC	DOSAGE	FORM
Metoclopramide	10mg	pill
	5–10mg	injection
Chlorpromazine	10mg	pill
	50mg	suppository
	25mg	injection
Prochlorperazine	10mg	pill
	25mg	suppository
	10mg	injection
Promethazine	25–50mg	pill
	25–50mg	suppository
	50–75mg	injection
Hydroxyzine	25–50mg	capsules
	75mg	injection

Sample migraine attack treatment plan

This sample plan shows how you can "step up" your treatment of a migraine attack if one particular combination of treatments fails. Use the combination that works best for you; different migraine attacks may need different combinations of medications. If you are not headache-free 4 hours after your migraine attack started, contact your doctor.

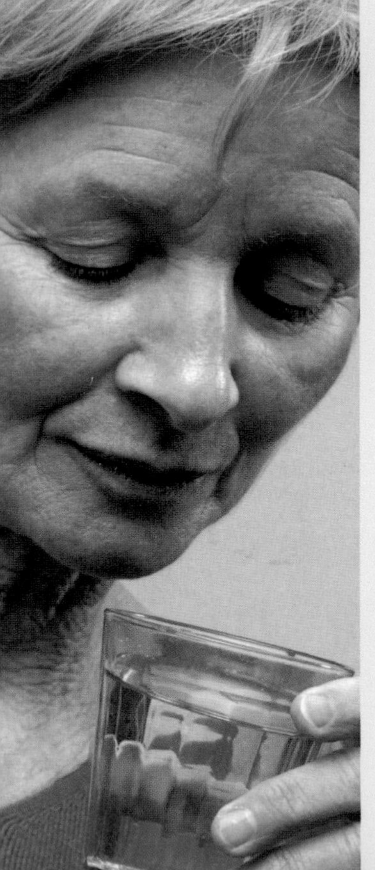

STEP 1: ONSET OF MIGRAINE

Immediately at onset of migraine attack:

- Drink 8 fluid ounces of water
- Stop what you are doing and find somewhere quiet, dark, and free of excess stimulation to rest until you are headache-free.
- Eat one serving each of carbohydrate and protein
- Take abortive medication: NSAID (N) and/or triptan (T), or NSAID with metoclopramide

Your medication: N .... dose .... route (oral)

Your medication: T .... dose .... route (oral)

If you are not headache-free 2 hours after commencing Step 1, you may need to "step up" treatment of your migraine attack. Move on to Step 2 of this migraine treatment plan.

STEP 2: IF MIGRAINE PERSISTS

- Drink 8 fluid ounces of water
- Eat one serving each of carbohydrate and protein
- Take abortive medication: same NSAID (N) and same triptan (T) plus adjunctive antiemetic (A)
- Sleep

Your medication: N .... dose .... route (oral)

Your medication: T .... dose .... route (oral)

Your medication: A .... dose .... route (oral)

Your medication: N .... dose .... route (oral)

Your medication: T .... dose .... route (nasal)

Your medication: A .... dose .... route (suppository)

Your medication: N .... dose .... route (injection)

Your medication: T .... dose .... route (injection)

Your medication: A .... dose .... route (suppository)

Your medication: N .... dose .... route (suppository)

Your medication: T .... dose .... route (nasal)

Your medication: A .... dose .... route (suppository)

Your medication: N .... dose .... route (injection)

Your medication: T .... dose .... route (injection)

Your medication: A .... dose .... route (injection)

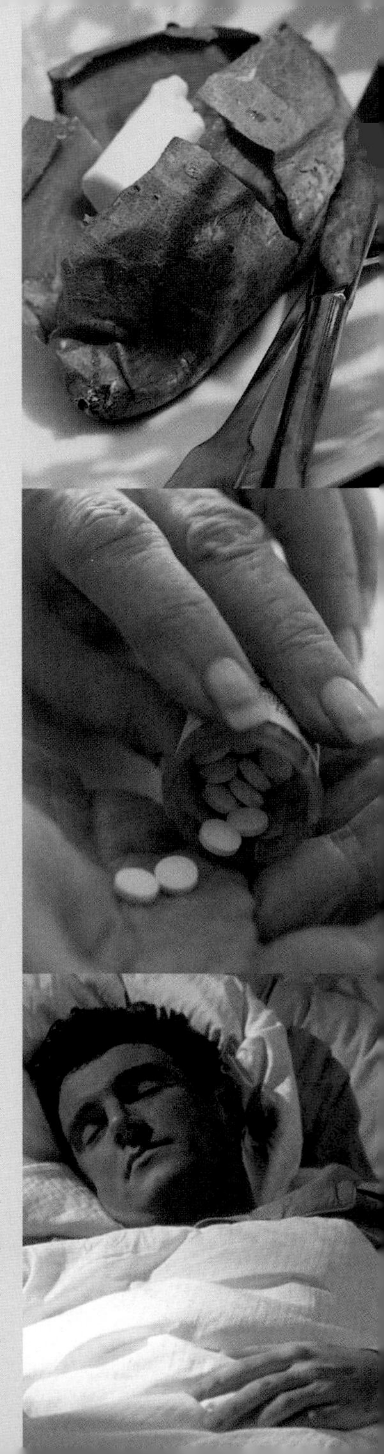

Emergencies

Q Do I need to go to the emergency room when I have a severe attack?

Few people who have suffered severe migraine attacks will be able to imagine anything much worse than going to a hospital's emergency department with a migraine. Waiting for hours to be seen in a noisy, stressful environment, and then being given drugs that are only going to make the migraine recur the next day is unlikely to offer much in the way of relief. A much better option for very severe attacks is abortive therapy using suppositories and injectable medications, which your doctor can provide.

Q How can suppositories and injectable medications keep me out of the emergency room?

Once a migraine attack progresses past the 2-hour point, gastric stasis (see p107) and central sensitization (see p27) make it very difficult to stop the attack. The quicker you get the effective dose of medication, the more successful you will be in aborting the attack. A rectal suppository or injection provides rapid delivery of medication into the blood when a migraine attack is not aborted with oral medication in the first 2 hours.

Q Can I give myself an injection?

Of course you can; diabetic patients and women undergoing fertility treatments are taught how to self-inject their medications. You need to discuss the use of injectable medications for abortive migraine treatment with your doctor. One of the triptans (sumatriptan) is available in an autoinjector and is very helpful for severe migraine attacks. The other injectable medications must be given by a traditional injection, but if your doctor agrees, you can learn how to give yourself your own "shot."

Complementary and psychological therapies

Q Are there complementary therapies for treatment of migraine attacks?

Yes. Many complementary therapies (such as relaxation techniques or massage), if initiated early in a mild attack, can defer the use of medication. It is important for many reasons to reduce the use of abortive medications, but if you delay treatment too long, more medication will be needed. In addition, the longer you have a migraine attack the more attacks you will have. If you want to cut back on the use of medication, you will need to treat attacks early and use nonmedication treatments to prevent attacks.

Q Is it true that the herb called feverfew can help with migraine?

Yes, feverfew can abort an attack (see p97). It is a herbal supplement with the same properties as nonsteroidal anti-inflammatory drugs (NSAIDs). As with NSAIDs, avoid feverfew if you have a stomach ulcer or gastrointestinal problems. Feverfew should not be used in combination with NSAIDs since this could have a cumulative effect.

Q How does my migraine prevention help me abort an attack?

The prevention of migraine attacks reduces the severity and duration of individual attacks as well as their frequency. When migraine attacks are less severe, they are easier to stop with abortive therapy. Maintaining an aggressive migraine prevention program with daily exercise and relaxation, stress management, and dietary restrictions can reduce the severity and frequency of attacks to the point where they can be aborted without medication.

Q How do I know when alternative abortive therapy is not working and I need medication?

This is a very important question. The answer is time. You can try complementary therapy for the migraine attack, but if you get no relief within 20 minutes you must proceed with medication. The longer you wait, the more difficult it will become to stop the attack. A migraine attack is caused by disturbances in brain function that progress over time. When medication is taken early in this process you are more likely to become pain-free within 2 hours. The longer a migraine attack continues past the 2-hour mark, the more likely you are to have another attack.

Q Can biofeedback training and relaxation techniques help prevent a migraine attack?

Yes, biofeedback, relaxation techniques, and even hypnosis can help prevent migraine attacks and, for some people, abort individual attacks. These techniques cause the release of natural painkillers called endorphins that relieve the headache and relax tense muscles. The goal of all relaxation techniques is to help you relax all your tense muscles. Once you learn some of these techniques, you can use them as part of abortive migraine attack therapy.

Q Will acupuncture help with my migraine attacks?

Acupuncture can be very helpful for both migraine prevention and relieving the muscle tension associated with an acute attack. Although it is not well understood how acupuncture works, it is thought to cause the release of natural painkillers called endorphins. Acupuncture is probably most effective when it is used as part of a comprehensive treatment approach. Indeed, this could be said about all treatment approaches: the most successful treatment programs are comprehensive, bringing the best parts of each treatment approach together to help you successfully treat your migraine.

Q How can psychological therapies help with a migraine attack?

The middle of a migraine attack is probably not the best time to dive into deep-seated emotional or mental problems—but there is much more to psychology than this. Techniques such as cognitive-behavioral therapy (CBT) offer practical ways to avoid anxiety and break free from negative patterns of thinking. The professionals available to help us with our psychological, social, and/or spiritual health have a wealth of knowledge and are trained in techniques that can reduce stress and increase relaxation, and therefore help abort a migraine attack.

Q How does the way I think prevent me from aborting a migraine attack?

Irritability and anxiety are biological symptoms of a migraine attack. Once the attack begins, anxious thoughts can escalate the migraine by causing excitation of the biological stress response system. For many people with migraine, the thought of another attack can be quite fearful. The possibility that the migraine attack will disrupt your day or, worse, bring your day to a halt is very frustrating. The more frustration you feel, the more you fuel the attack. Searching out professional help to learn coping strategies can reduce the anxiety and frustration that is associated with a migraine attack.

Q How can I reduce the muscle tension caused by the migraine attacks?

Nonpharmacological methods of treating migraine attacks become important when the frequency of attacks increases. These methods include the use of TENS units, heat or cold application, and relaxation techniques. TENS units are medical devices applied to the skin that deliver stimulating impulses to muscles, causing tense muscles to relax. People who have significant muscle tension with their migraine may benefit from massage therapy and/or physical therapy.

Q Will I need to seek the help of a professional to reduce the muscle tension?

If you experience significant muscle tension with your migraine attacks, you will need the help of an appropriate professional. Dental splints may help those who have facial muscle tightness. There is a significant overlap between people who have migraine and those with temporomandibular joint dysfunction (misalignment of the jaw bones, causing face pain). An ergonomic analysis of your work-related posture and movements might help alleviate the muscle tension associated with attacks. Discussion with a physical therapist regarding your work setting and activities may help you to identify mechanical triggers for attacks and factors that aggravate attacks.

Q Can rubbing a cream or ointment directly on the forehead work to stop a headache?

The application of herbal or nonpharmacological creams or ointments may or may not help a migraine attack. Before using them you should ask your doctor whether they can be absorbed through your skin and thus possibly cause a drug interaction with your other medications. If you find that rubbing a cream or ointment on your forehead helps abort your migraine and you feel it is worth the money, then there is no reason not to use it.

Q Can chiropractic or osteopathic treatment abort a migraine attack?

Yes. The techniques used by chiropractors or osteopaths can sometimes be particularly useful when your migraine has progressed for hours or days and developed into central sensitization (see p27), and you are experiencing neck pain and muscle tension. This type of manipulative therapy can be effective in relieving neck pain and muscle tension. However, you should be evaluated by your doctor for neck problems that could be made worse by such techniques before you start this type of treatment program.

Exercise and sleep

Q Can I exercise when I have a migraine attack?

You must be sure you have completely aborted the attack before you exercise, and you should decrease the intensity of your workout. You must be well hydrated and avoid hypoglycemia (low blood sugar). You may want to forego your usual workout and take a relaxing walk instead.

Q Can I still exercise if I have had to repeat my medication?

Do not exercise if you have not been able to abort your migraine attack within 2 hours. If the attack was so severe that it required a second dose of medication, exercise could trigger a recurrence of the attack. If you used a sedating antiemetic with your repeat medication it would be risky to exercise—you need to rest. You can return to your exercise routine the next day, but reduce the intensity.

Q How can I avoid getting away from my exercise routine once I have had a migraine attack?

Having missed a day or two of exercise due to migraine, you might find it difficult to get back to your routine. Try to do this slowly. The important thing is to do something each day and gradually increase the intensity of your exercise. You must avoid dehydration and hypoglycemia (low blood sugar) during exercise since you will be more vulnerable to another attack in the days following one.

Q Can my sleep patterns affect my migraine attacks?

Irregular sleep habits can trigger migraine attacks. The problem arises when sedating medications have made you sleep all day, and you cannot sleep at night. Another problem is the insomnia that may occur the night before an attack. If you can't fall asleep, try using relaxation techniques. You may use antiemetics for sedation, but do not use sedatives, which could trigger another attack.

Managing time

Q How do I avoid losing time as a result of migraine attacks?

Unfortunately, there is no way to avoid giving up time to a migraine attack. If you do not take the time needed to treat migraine attacks adequately, they will only increase in frequency and steal more of your time. Too many headache sufferers push through their migraine attacks, allowing the headaches and associated symptoms to decrease their productivity. A migraine attack is more than just a headache. The associated symptoms that adversely affect your ability to concentrate and your mood diminish your quality of life. The only way to avoid lost time to migraine attacks is to prevent the attacks.

Q After a migraine, I often try to make up for lost time. Can this trigger another attack?

In the first day or so following a migraine attack, you are more vulnerable to another attack. Rather than over-committing yourself the day after a migraine attack, you need to lighten your workload. If you overdo things, you will simply risk triggering another attack and fall even further behind in your work.

Q What if I cannot take the time to treat a migraine attack?

If you continue to push yourself through a migraine attack, you will increase the duration of the attack. By not completely aborting migraine attacks, you cause progression of the disease that leads to chronic daily headache. You may need to ask for help or transfer some of your responsibilities intermittently. This should not be necessary often, since with appropriate preventive therapy most of your migraine attacks should be easily treated with one dose of medication.

Q How important is it that I track my migraine attacks?

Once you have completely aborted your migraine attack it is important that you document the attack in your headache diary (see p86). You will need to review the 2 or 3 days before the attack to try to identify possible triggers, such as foods or beverages you have consumed. By reviewing the circumstances surrounding the migraine attack you will be able to make lifestyle changes that can prevent the next attack. Your migraine diary will give you an accurate assessment of your migraine control. Once you have identified a problem with migraine control by seeing more frequent attacks documented in your diary, you can return to your doctor for adjustments in your medications.

Q How can the migraine diary influence my medication management?

Individual migraine attacks vary, and attack frequency can also vary over time. By accurately documenting the frequency, intensity, duration, and timing of your migraine attacks, you and your doctor can determine the most effective medication regimen for you.

Q Will the use of a migraine diary help me monitor my medication intake and side effects?

One of the most tedious aspects of dealing with a chronic illness is taking medications. The difficulty arises when you do not take enough or overmedicate. Migraine is a treatable chronic illness, but for treatment to be effective you must take your medication correctly. If you aggressively treat migraine you will not have to deal with medications that often. When you have a migraine attack it is very important that you document what medications you took, how much, the side effects if any, and the treatment results. By documenting your treatment results in your migraine diary, you will be able to assess the effectiveness of your medications more objectively.

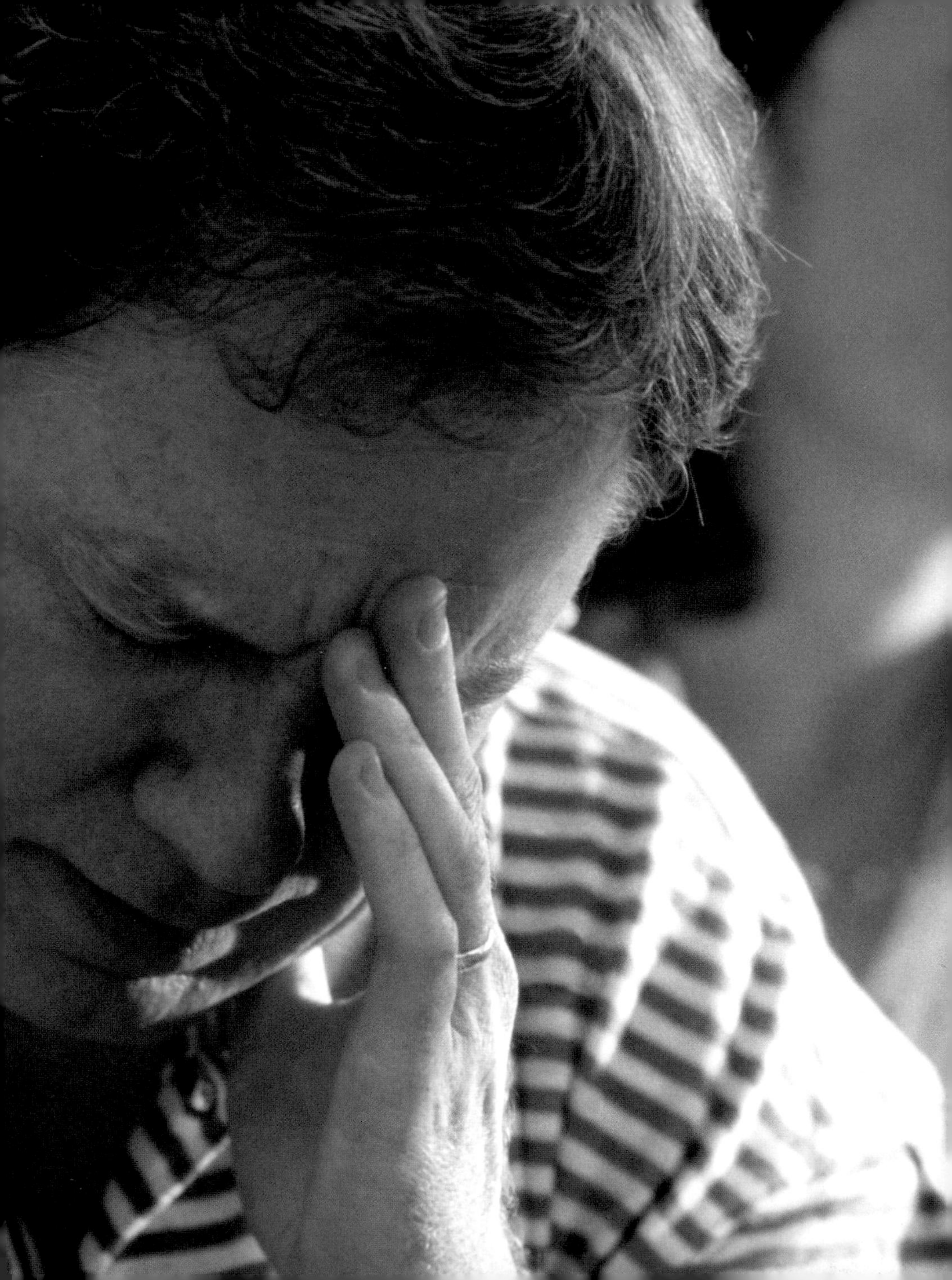

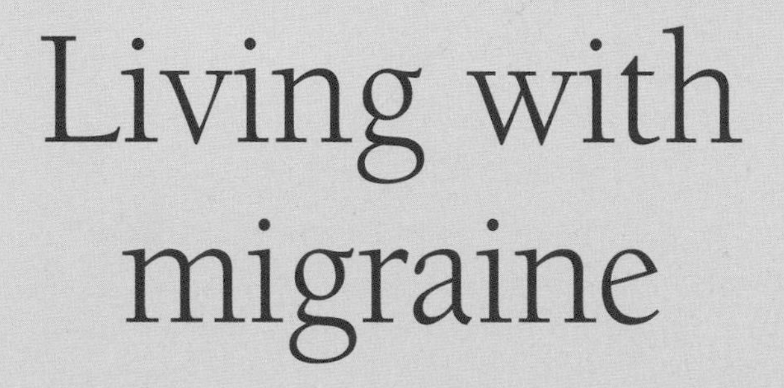

Living with migraine

With a better understanding of your disease, you can sort out the problems you might face while living with migraine. If you take steps to reduce stress, make proper plans, and enlist the help of others, then you will find it less difficult to accommodate a comprehensive migraine treatment program into your life. Once you successfully gain control of your migraine attacks, you will see the benefits of all your hard work.

Changing your attitude

Q Every time I have an attack, I tell myself I need to do something about my migraine but then I never do. How can I get motivated to take action?

You are not alone. Many people put off doing anything about their migraine until it becomes so bad that it starts to interfere with their lives. Migraine can be simple to treat with early intervention, but unfortunately the longer you go without treatment, the more you will need to do to gain control of your illness. In addition, the longer you delay treatment the more time you will lose to unnecessary pain and suffering. Making a decision not to allow migraine to take over another day of your life should be all the motivation you need to get started on the path to headache-free days.

Q When I think about changing my lifestyle I feel overwhelmed. How do I get started?

Lifestyle changes with any chronic illness can be overwhelming. The more you understand migraine, the easier it will be to make these changes. The key to success is to start with a plan. Allow time for relaxation and exercise. Begin your dietary changes by reviewing your current eating habits, and then start to eliminate foods that trigger migraine. Finally, identify the areas that are creating stress and begin to solve the relevant problems.

Q I find myself being fearful of the next migraine attack. How can I become more confident?

You need to give yourself and the treatment program time to work. Success breeds success. A comprehensive treatment program will reduce the frequency and severity of your migraine attacks. In time, you will become more confident that you can prevent attacks and control those you do have. Stay dedicated to your treatment program, document your success in your migraine diary, and have patience. It takes time to treat such a chronic illness.

Q Avoiding food triggers makes sense, but it is so difficult. Will I always have to avoid them?

The extent to which you need to restrict intake of certain foods or beverages depends on the frequency of your attacks and your circumstances. If you have frequent attacks and need preventive migraine medications, then restricting dietary triggers and reducing stress is crucial for the best outcome. On the other hand, if migraine attacks are infrequent, then an occasional food trigger will be less likely to trigger an attack. Beware: consuming a food trigger when other migraine triggers are present may be all it takes to push you over the edge into a severe attack.

Q I seem to do well until something unexpected happens and then I have a migraine attack. What can I do to avoid a migraine?

You cannot anticipate every possible situation that could trigger a migraine, so the best defense against a migraine attack is to have your illness as well controlled as possible. Migraine is an illness of the stress response system; therefore, whenever you are under stress you are more vulnerable to an attack. It is important that you maintain your treatment program during stressful circumstances. You need to continue your exercise and relaxation routine, get adequate rest, and stick with your migraine diet.

Q People are a pain; they give me a headache. How do I avoid the stress caused by dealing with people?

There is no doubt that some people can be a real challenge. The first step is to remind yourself not to waste your serotonin (a calming brain chemical) on people who annoy you. When you become upset or frustrated with someone, your brain releases epinephrine (an activating brain chemical), which can trigger a migraine attack. The key is to limit your interaction and decide how much effort you want to invest in the relationship. If the relationship is important, then you may need a third party to help find a resolution.

The benefits of planning

Q I have started my migraine diet but I am getting bored with my food. How can I make my diet more interesting?

Your treatment program will not be successful if you do not plan for it. Unless you think ahead, plan your menus, and prepare a shopping list, you will find yourself eating the same thing everyday. The migraine diet is not that different from a healthy diet. However, it does take away the convenience of packaged food and eating out all the time.You may want to visit your local bookstore for cookbooks. You can find new recipes to try. Some of the recipes may require some changes to make them headache-friendly.

Q I find it difficult to say "no" to my family or friends when they offer me food that I need to avoid. What can I do?

You must learn to say "no, thank you." Many people express their love by offering food. When you say no they feel rejected, so it is very important to be nice. When someone offers you food, it is not the time to go into a long drawn-out explanation about migraine and food triggers. Simply say "no, thank you" with a gracious attitude. If you find someone insisting that you eat a food that you know is a trigger, then you may need to tell him or her politely that you must avoid certain foods because of migraine.

Q I can stick with my program until I have a headache. How do I get back to my routine after a headache?

You need to have a post-headache day plan. The day following a migraine attack, you must adhere strictly to your migraine diet, reduce the intensity of your exercise routine, and avoid trying to make up for lost time. Review your daily responsibilities. Eliminate unnecessary activities, defer chores to someone else if you can, and do only what you can easily manage.

Q My day planner is full as it is, so how am I going to add migraine treatment to it?

You need to decide that adding your migraine treatment to your day planner is worth the effort. The fact is that either you add migraine treatment to your planner or migraine will add a headache to your day. You need to make time for a daily exercise program and daily relaxation. Making time for shopping is essential to ensure you have food for your special dietary needs. Once you have better control over your migraine, you will have plenty of room on your planner, because you will be able to use your time more efficiently.

Q How do I stick to my exercise and relaxation routine no matter what?

First, you need to understand that it is impossible to maintain a strict exercise and relaxation program all the time. You need to plan for your daily exercise and relaxation, but there will be times when life keeps you from your routine. When your routine is interrupted, make every effort to get back on track as soon as possible. Depending upon the circumstances, you may have to reduce the time for your program. Once things are back to normal, you can dedicate yourself to your full relaxation and exercise routine.

Q What can I do to make my plan succeed?

Taking the time to write down your treatment plan will help you succeed with your treatment program. A written plan will help you remember to do your relaxation and exercise program. Reviewing your treatment and menu plans will help you to assess your progress in changing your lifestyle. You will be able to see your areas of success and identify those that need a little extra work. In the beginning, set realistic goals for yourself, then as time goes on you can make bigger changes.

Myth "No one understands or cares about my migraine"

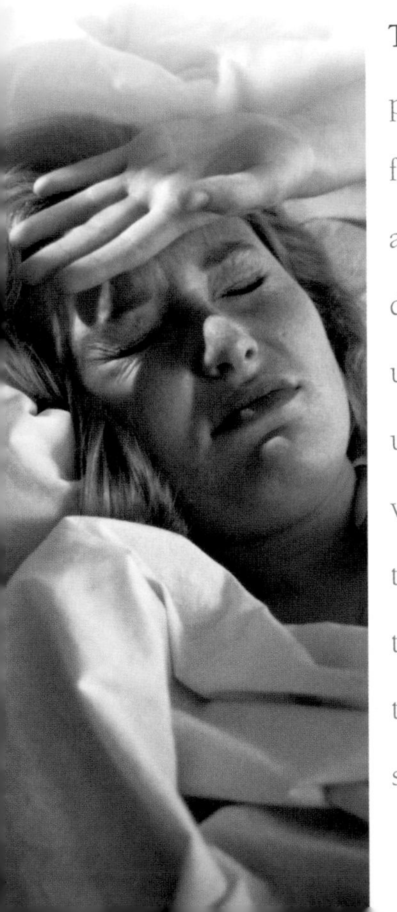

Truth Suffering from migraine while the people around you are healthy and headache-free can seem very lonely; however, you are not alone. In the last decade or so, there have been dramatic advancements in the treatment and understanding of this chronic illness. Those of us who have dedicated our lives to helping people with migraine are passionate about making sure that sufferers know that there is treatment for their disease. We want not only to help alleviate the pain of the attack but also to eliminate the stigma of the illness.

How other people can help

Q How do I find out more about migraine?

Learning more about migraine and keeping up to date on new information is very helpful. There are many resources that can help you with migraine education. You can do research at your local library or at a medical library. Information is also available in bookstores and on the internet. Your doctor may have educational information. Pharmaceutical companies provide educational material and website information about migraine as well.

Q Who can I turn to for help?

The first person to turn to is your doctor. Many people suffer for years without talking to their doctor. Depending upon your situation, you may need to see other healthcare providers too. Many professionals can help you with stress management, physical therapy, physical fitness, and dietary counseling. Initially, it may take time to organize a treatment team and you may need to consult different professionals before you find the right people, but your doctor should be your first point of contact.

Q How can I find others who have migraine?

Migraine is very common. It will not take you long to discover other sufferers once you start your treatment program. You will find that people with migraine are very interested in your experiences and treatment. On finding others, you may want to form home groups or devise ways to come together to share ideas. Most communities have organized support groups as well. You can get information about such support groups and migraine associations by contacting the organizations listed in the Useful addresses section (see p184).

Q How can I find the time to do the research and planning needed to manage my migraine?

That is a problem we all could handle a little better. Modern-day lifestyles force us to want more and work more, making it very difficult to fit everything into a 24-hour day. A quick trip to the bookstore for a book on time management may be very helpful. There are many reasons why people overcommit themselves. You may need to seek the help of a professional if you are unable to make time for your migraine treatment.

Q Can someone help me deal with the financial burden of changing my lifestyle?

Healthcare costs and insurance issues can be a real financial burden for many people. Learning more about your insurance coverage will help you lower the cost of your medical care. Prevention can reduce the cost by reducing the amount of money spent on abortive therapy. You will also increase your income as you reduce the amount of time lost from work because of migraine attacks. By not eating out, you will save even more. You may need to take the time to prepare a budget that allows for your migraine care. Discussing your financial situation with a social worker or financial advisor may help you prepare a budget.

Q How do I manage when I have a severe migraine attack?

People who have migraine are often very independent, and they may feel that asking for help is worse than the attack itself. Whether you like it or not, there will be a time during a severe migraine when you will need help. You may need someone to drive you home or to the doctor, or to pick up medication from the pharmacy. There are times you may need help with home or work responsibilities. You need to plan for such circumstances. Identify a few individuals you can turn to for help during an attack. You can always return the favor when they need you.

Reducing stress at home

Q I get very stressed when I try to take care of myself and everything else I have to do at home. How can I do it all?

Accommodating your treatment program and home responsibilities can be a real source of stress. As you continue with your lifestyle changes and succeed with better migraine control, you will find this challenge less overwhelming. Often the stress is created by your need to take care of everything yourself. Trying to continue your lifestyle as usual and adding your treatment program will only cause unnecessary stress. If you hope to succeed with your treatment, you will need to make some adjustments in your lifestyle to accommodate your migraine care.

Q I feel guilty when I cannot do things with my family and friends. How do I find time for social activities, as well as my treatment program?

In the beginning, you may need to make some changes in your usual activities to allow time for your migraine treatment program. Placing some of your activities on hold until you have your migraine under control will reduce stress. The necessary commitments can be shared with family or friends. Before you involve yourself in an activity, make sure you can maintain your treatment-friendly lifestyle.

Q Should I ask my family to adapt their schedule because of my treatment?

Yes, one family member's chronic illness is a burden that the entire family must help them to bear. Unless migraine is aggressively treated, the attacks can cause considerable disruption for everybody around you. If changing your family's schedule helps reduce the frequency of attacks, it will benefit everyone. Your family can, and should, support you, so do not feel guilty about asking them to contribute to the success of your treatment program.

Q How can I identify relationships or financial issues that are creating stress?

Stress increases the frequency of migraine attacks. In order to reduce stress, you need to determine what issues are creating problems. Relationships and financial situations are common sources of stress for many people. Monitoring your migraine attacks, tracking them in your migraine diary, and documenting stressful events will help you identify sources of stress. When you are able to determine the sources of your stress, you are better able to formulate a plan to deal with the problem.

Q Can my home environment cause stress?

Yes, your domestic environment certainly can cause stress and trigger a migraine attack. Your home needs to be migraine-friendly. Making sure you have a quiet, comfortable setting to go to when you have a migraine attack is an important aspect of your abortive therapy. Reducing glare and eliminating pungent odors and unnecessary noise will help decrease migraine triggers. Maintaining a home environment that is both relaxing and turmoil-free will go a long way in helping you prevent migraine.

Q When I listen to the news I become very upset. How can I prevent global issues from causing me overwhelming stress?

We live in a time when 24-hour news channels provide us with constant updates on wars, natural disasters, humanitarian crises, and global warming. Obviously, it is important that you stay informed. However, you need to avoid overexposure to stressful news. Therefore, you should limit the amount of time you spend listening to news about events that could upset you. If you are feeling overwhelmed, find someone with whom you can share your concerns, or seek professional help for stress management.

Household planning

Q How can I involve my family in my migraine care?

Involving family members in planning and shopping for your migraine-friendly diet will give everyone an opportunity to spend time together. It will also ensure that everyone finds foods they enjoy. Preparing meals together will reduce stress; the rest of your family do not have to avoid all the foods that you need to, but they can help by not eating these around you. Everyone can benefit from a routine exercise program as well. Spending time together during exercise is healthy, bonding, and can encourage you and help you maintain your routine.

Q How do I match my migraine treatment to my family's lifestyle?

This requires planning. By reviewing the family calendar in advance, you will be able to integrate your treatment schedule with their activities. Initially, everyone will need to make some sacrifices to help you accommodate your treatment plan. By sharing information about migraine, you will help your family understand the changes needed to make your treatment a success. In time, they will see the difference their sacrifices have made and will come to enjoy your headache-free time as much as you do.

Q How do I manage the stress of household responsibilities?

Ask your family to help with the various household responsibilities; this will give you an opportunity to do your relaxation techniques and will reduce stress. You may want to have a family meeting to discuss household chores and to develop a plan. By assigning chores, you can eliminate the stress of trying to do everything by yourself. If you live alone you may need to ask friends or family members to help you.

Q I am able to control my migraine attacks until the weather changes. Is there anything I can do during such times?

When there are uncontrollable migraine triggers such as weather, season, or hormonal changes, you need to be especially careful to follow your treatment plan rigorously. You must continue with your exercise and relaxation program, and it is very important that you avoid fatigue and all other triggers during these times.

Q How important is it that I have a written treatment plan with stated goals?

When you formulate a treatment plan with identified goals and objectives, you will be able to assess your progress. You can review it every week to determine if any changes are needed. If you find areas that are causing difficulty, then you can seek help. Your plan needs to remain flexible since life circumstances are always changing.

Q How do I manage my dietary changes with everything else I have to do?

Initially you will need to plan your menus in advance. You can use them to make a shopping list. By planning menus, you can avoid migraine triggers and save time by shopping for food in advance. You will need to invest time in making dietary changes, but the return will be more migraine-free time.

Q How do I make time for exercise and relaxation?

Make a commitment each day to spend time, even a short period, on exercise and relaxation. It is important that you establish a daily habit. Once your routine is set, you can increase the time. The key to success is consistency. You will need to stay dedicated to your treatment program.

Q How do I convince others that my treatment program is important?

Unfortunately, you may not be able to convince everyone that exercise, relaxation, and "special food" is necessary for treating your migraine. This can be frustrating, but if people simply refuse to recognize that migraine is a "real" disease, you may be better off saving your energy.

Helping other people with migraine

Q How can I convince my mother that her analgesics are causing her headaches?

You may find it difficult to convince your mother that she is having a medication overuse headache. You can provide her with information about migraine and the different treatment options, and give her the names of headache specialists in your area. Encourage her to seek help by pointing out that she will have the opportunity to experience more headache-free days.

Q How can I help my friend when she has a severe migraine attack?

It is very important that people who are having a migraine attack stop what they are doing and take their medications. You can assist your friend by offering to help with home responsibilities, such as preparing meals, or work commitments. She may need help with transportation, child care, or shopping as well. Often, knowing they have someone to depend upon during an attack can be helpful to people in reducing stress.

Q My husband has severe migraine but he will not do anything about it. What can I do?

Your husband may be like many people who wait for their migraine to go away. You need to be gentle in sharing information with him about migraine. If he is having a severe attack, it is not the ideal time to remind him that he needs to do something about his migraine. What you can do is help him reduce stress, perhaps by participating in an exercise program with him, and provide more migraine-friendly food choices. When he is feeling well, encourage him to learn more about migraine.

Q My friend has migraine. How can I help her with her treatment?

People who have migraine are very appreciative when friends and family express an interest in helping them with their illness. You can help your friend in many ways. You can offer to help with her daily chores, shopping, or errands. You can offer to prepare migraine-friendly dishes or suggest that you exercise with your friend. Most of all, having someone who understands the problems goes a long way in helping a person deal with his or her new lifestyle.

Q What should I do when my wife has a migraine attack?

Those who live with people at risk of migraine attacks can encourage them to start treatment as soon as an attack starts. Encourage your wife to stop what she is doing and use her abortive therapy. While she rests, prepare a snack and offer her water; eating and drinking will help abort the migraine attack. Make the environment migraine-friendly by reducing glare and noise. If the attack has not been completely aborted in 2 hours, encourage your wife to treat it again. The day after a migraine attack, offer assistance because it is important that she does not overexert herself.

Q My 10-year-old daughter has migraine. How do I deal with her school?

You need to communicate with the school officials about your daughter's chronic illness. Having written instructions regarding diet, hydration, and physical activity will help teachers understand your child's special healthcare requirements. It is important that you provide the school nurse with medications and instructions for abortive therapy. Emphasize the importance of early treatment for a migraine attack. If the attack is not completely aborted within a couple of hours, the school needs to send the child home for repeat medication and rest.

Managing your medication

Q I fast intermittently for reasons of faith. Can I take my abortive therapy without food?

Fasting may trigger a migraine attack. Abortive therapy is more effective once dehydration and hypoglycemia (low blood sugar) are treated. However, if you must fast, you can take your medications without food. Watch out for a stomach upset if NSAIDs are taken without food.

Q My migraine attacks are infrequent. Do I always have to carry my abortive medication with me?

When migraine attacks are infrequent, it is easy to be caught off guard without your abortive medications. An attack can occur at any time, so you must be prepared to treat it early. Lack of medication will delay treatment and make the attack more difficult to treat.

Q Can I adjust my preventive medication dosage?

You should consult your doctor if you think your preventive medication dosage needs to be changed. He or she may at first prescribe a small dose, instructing you to increase it gradually as you tolerate the side effects.

Q What happens if I miss doses or run out of my preventive medication?

You can trigger a migraine attack by missing doses of your medication, so it is important to take them as instructed. Pill containers that provide sections for each day of the week may help you remember each dose.

Q If I develop side effects, should I stop my preventive medication?

You should consult your doctor. Some drug side effects are serious and require that the medication be discontinued. Others may be less serious and only require a change in dosage. Some preventive migraine medications can cause problems if discontinued suddenly; therefore you need to talk to your doctor before you stop taking a drug.

Dealing with work

Q What can I do to minimize my chances of having a migraine attack at work?

You can avoid a migraine attack at work by reducing the number of triggers you are exposed to as much as possible. You may need to change your physical setting to alleviate muscle strain and glare. You need to avoid dietary triggers, such as dehydration and hypoglycemia, so make sure you drink enough fluids and eat regularly while you are at work. Try to avoid migraine food triggers; you may need to bring suitable food from home. Finally, you need to reduce work-related stress.

Q How can I make the meals I eat at work more migraine-friendly?

Preparing food to take to work may involve extra planning. You can save time by making extra servings for dinner the night before, then take those to work for lunch. Preparing several lunches beforehand may be helpful. You can eat out for lunch; however, you will need to avoid food additives and food triggers as much as possible. Even if you do eat out for lunch, you will need to take your midmorning and afternoon snacks with you to work. Making these changes may seem overwhelming at first, but when you start to experience fewer headaches, it will be worth it.

Q What can I do to relieve stress while I am at work?

Taking a break from your work for a few minutes every hour can help relieve stress. A short walk can be helpful, or you may want to learn a relaxation exercise you can do at your desk. If necessary, discuss with your employer your need to take a short break and have your snack. You can explain that by preventing a migraine attack you will be more productive and avoid lost work time.

Q I am concerned about my employer's and coworkers' reactions if I tell them I have migraine. What if they think I do not measure up to the pressures of my job?

Unfortunately, many people do have the belief that people who have migraine are somehow weak and cannot measure up to the pressures of life. This idea could not be further from the truth. Most people with migraine are hardworking, loyal employees who care greatly about their job performance. Educating employers and coworkers may require tact and time. When presenting your situation, approach the issue from their point of view, not yours. You need to demonstrate to them how your health will benefit your workplace and your employer.

Q What can I do to reduce or eliminate work-related stress?

The first step in reducing work-related stress is to leave work at your workplace. Bringing work home with you creates stress. If you are unable to complete your assigned work, then you may need to discuss your workload with your employer. Difficulties with coworkers can be another source of stress in the workplace. You need to address any problems that are creating strife at work. Strained work relationships will affect your productivity and make you more vulnerable to migraine attacks.

Q How do I deal with time off work because of my migraine?

Missing work for medical care or a migraine attack is inevitable. You can discuss your need to be away from work with your employer. Familiarize yourself with the office policies on sick leave or personal time. You can explain to your employer that, with time and if properly treated, migraine can be easily controlled. Explain that by getting appropriate treatment, you will spend more time working even if you have a migraine attack and that it will also reduce the number of work days lost.

Myth "Migraine attacks are inevitable during vacations because of stress"

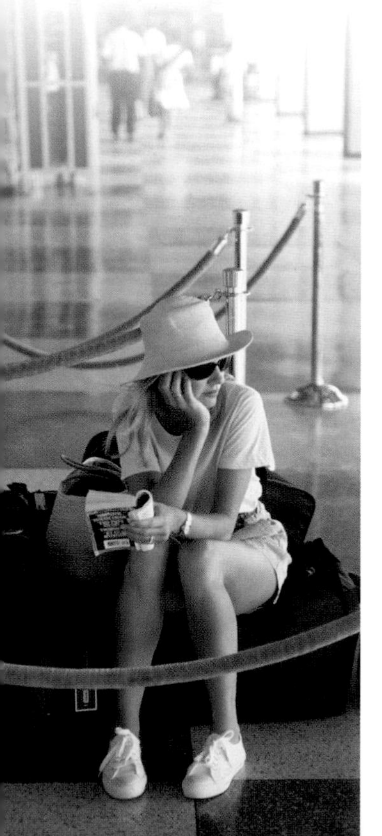

Truth Vacations can be very stressful: you are in a different environment, dealing with new people, and often spending more money than usual and trying new activities. However, there are ways to reduce vacation stress and minimize the threat of an attack. The key is to do less, not more. The best thing about a vacation is rest; take advantage of this time to relax and let your brain make serotonin, not waste it.

Travel and holidays

Q Why do I always have a migraine attack when I travel?

Travel creates a situation in which several potential triggers occur at the same time. There is the excitement and stress of the actual travel coupled with food triggers, possible altitude change, schedule change, and disrupted sleep patterns. Before your trip, anticipate as many triggers as possible. Plan your travel and make arrangements to avoid migraine triggers. By reducing the number of triggers, it is possible to avoid a migraine attack.

Q How do I travel with my medications?

Travel may create special circumstances that you need to consider regarding your medications. Most medications must stay at room temperature; therefore, you need to avoid extremes of hot or cold. For example, you should not place your medication in luggage that will be checked at the airport or stowed in the trunk of a car. You can travel with suppositories, but these need to be refrigerated once you arrive at your destination. Most importantly, do not forget to take your medications with you when you travel; place them beside your travel documents to remind you. Finally, stay calm and enjoy the trip.

Q I use injectable medications for my migraine. Can I take them onto a plane?

This depends on the level of security at the airport. Contact the airlines before your flight to find out what you can and cannot take onto the plane. You may need a note from your doctor. If you cannot travel with your injectable medications, then you and your doctor will need to alter your abortive therapy, or your doctor may be able to provide you with a prescription you can fill once you arrive at your destination.

Planning for a stress-free vacation

Vacations don't have to be stressful. We choose to make them stressful with our unrealistic expectations and overspending. No wonder we end up with a headache. To prevent a migraine attack, you must make sure you do not disturb your body's serotonin levels. You can do this by having a sensible travel and vacation plan. Make a decision to enjoy your vacation without a headache.

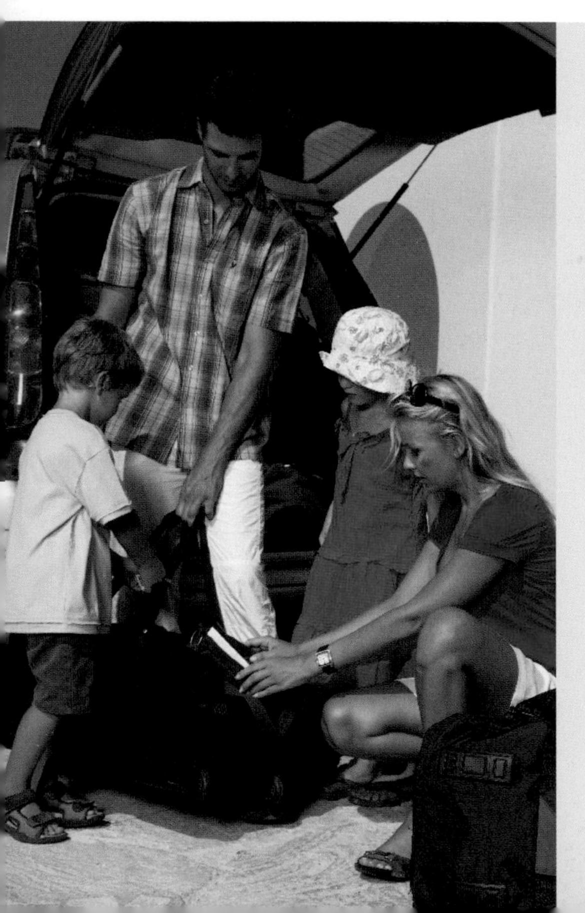

AVOIDING JET LAG

Air travel across several time zones disrupts the body's regular sleep-wake cycle and can trigger a migraine attack. The more time zones you cross, the more jet lag you are likely to experience. The key to avoiding jet lag and migraine attacks is to synchronize your body clock with local conditions. For a few days before you travel, get up and go to bed slightly earlier than normal, if flying east, or slightly later than normal if flying west. If you arrive at your destination in the morning, try to get plenty of bright, natural light to help you stay awake. If you arrive in the evening, go to bed at a reasonable time. Try to be as well rested as possible before the flight—being tired or stressed will not help your migraine. Eat light meals and drink plenty of water during the flight.

MAKING A TRAVEL AND VACATION PLAN

If you are going to avoid a migraine attack during travel or a vacation then you need to make a plan. A plan will help you reduce stress and ensure compliance with your migraine treatment. The following steps will help you with your travel or vacation plan.

What are your goals and expectations? Deciding what you want to achieve will help you stay realistic about your expectations. For example, do you want to relax, enjoy your time off, and spend time with your loved ones, or are you somehow expecting the perfect vacation with everyone miraculously changing into perfect people, getting everything they ever wanted?

What activities do you plan on doing? Choosing activities that you enjoy and can financially afford will help you plan realistically. Consider your timetable before planning your activities. You need to avoid the stress of doing too much and not having enough time for rest.

What factors can get in your way? You need to anticipate what might prevent you from adhering to your migraine treatment program. You will need time in your schedule for exercise and relaxation. Making arrangements for dietary needs are necessary if you want to avoid a migraine attack. You may need to shop for food and offer to help with food preparation.

What will you do if things do not go as you planned? Anticipate travel and vacation disruptions. You may not be able to plan for every possible stressful situation, but the important thing is that you remain calm. If you start to have a migraine attack, treat it immediately.

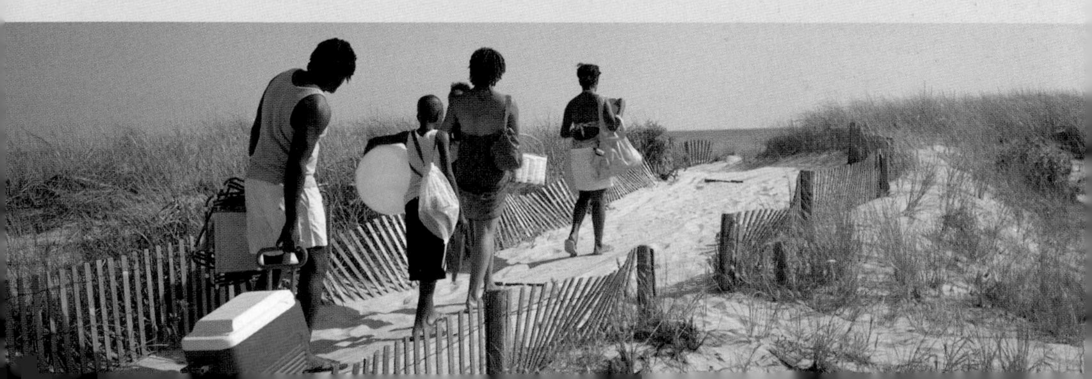

Driving and migraine

Q Can I drive a car or some other vehicle?

Being diagnosed with migraine does not prevent you from driving. However, the Federal Aviation Administration will not allow you to fly a plane. Migraine does not create any safety concerns while in control of a vehicle, unless you drive during a migraine attack or while taking medications that affect your ability to drive safely.

Q How can a migraine attack affect my driving?

During a migraine attack you can experience visual disturbances, vertigo (dizziness), and difficulty concentrating. If you were to drive while experiencing a migraine attack, these associated symptoms would make you vulnerable to driving errors and place you and others at risk of serious injury. If you begin to experience a migraine attack while driving, you should stop the vehicle and immediately treat the attack. You should not resume driving until you have completely aborted the attack and are sure that your medications will not interfere with your ability to drive.

Q Can my medications affect my ability to drive safely?

Many preventive medications do not affect your driving ability; however, some may. If your medication causes difficulty concentrating or drowsiness then you should not drive. Abortive medications do not typically affect judgment or cause drowsiness. If you are sure you have aborted a migraine attack, you will be able to drive unless you have used abortive medications that sedate. Alcohol can interact with prescription medication, so you need to avoid drinking alcoholic beverages.

Q Sometimes driving in busy traffic can trigger my migraine attacks. How can I avoid such attacks while I'm driving?

Driving can act as a trigger for a migraine attack because of the stress and fatigue involved, as well as glare and pungent odors. You can reduce your risk of a migraine attack while driving if you maintain the necessary dietary restrictions, take breaks from driving to relax and stretch out, avoid glare by wearing sunglasses, and avoid traveling behind vehicles emitting exhaust fumes. Try not to become too frustrated with the behavior of other drivers. Remaining calm will help you avoid a migraine attack.

Q How do I avoid driving when I have a migraine attack?

There are likely to be occasions when you cannot drive because of an acute migraine attack but you need to make a journey. Organize a few individuals who could help you with transportation when you have an attack, and discuss your requirements with them to make sure they would be available when you need them. You may find it difficult to ask for help but you must understand how dangerous it could be for you and others if you drive during an attack.

Q My family and I enjoy road trips. How can I avoid a migraine attack while we are on one of these trips?

If you follow the travel plan discussed previously, it will help reduce your risk of having a migraine attack while you're on the road. Eating out becomes a bit more of a challenge on a road trip. It is very important that you do your best to stay focused and do not relax your dietary restrictions. Review the previous discussion about driving and migraine triggers. You need to avoid long periods of driving time without stopping to walk around and relax. Try to reduce the stress of driving with children by making sure they are entertained with playing games or listening to music.

Eating out

When eating out, you need to plan on saying "no" to certain foods and be prepared to make the right food choices. Many restaurants offer healthier choices that can be migraine-friendly. Selecting your food with care can help you avoid a migraine attack. Your food choices should be as free from additives, such as soy, as possible. By avoiding creamy salad dressings, soups, sauces, and gravies, you reduce your risk of exposure to a migraine trigger. Keep your choices simple by choosing grilled entrées, steamed vegetables, and simple salads with an oil and white vinegar dressing.

MEAT DISHES

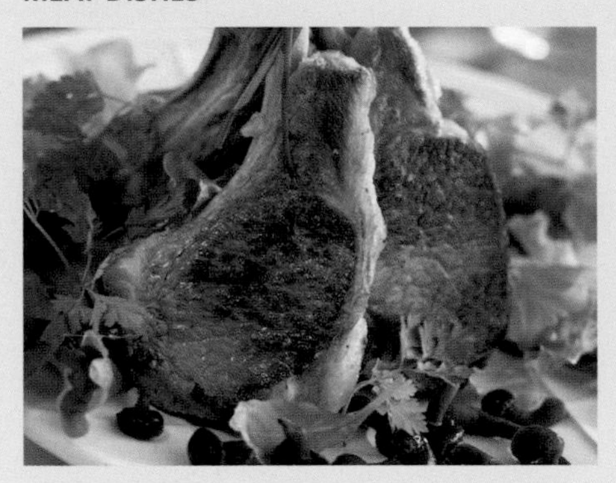

Good choices: Grilled chicken, steak, or lamb without sauce or tenderizers, served with steamed vegetables and a garden salad with oil and white vinegar dressing.

Bad choices: Breaded or deep fried chicken, barbequed ribs, "seasoned steaks" with onion rings, and salad with citrus and creamy dressing.

FISH DISHES

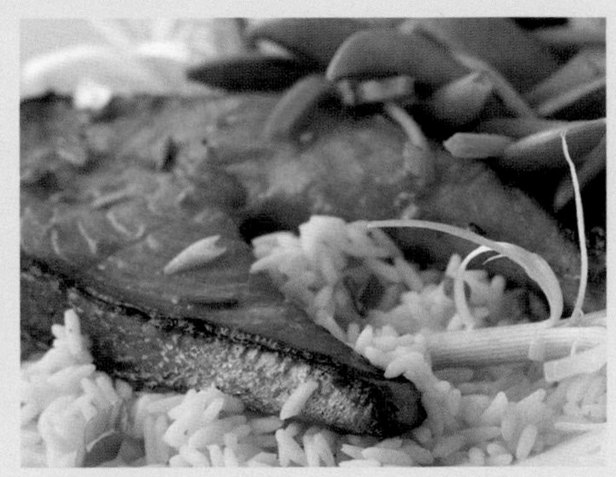

Good choices: Baked or poached salmon, mild white fish or tuna with plain rice, steamed broccoli and cauliflower. Tuna burgers, homemade fries, lettuce, and tomato.

Bad choices: Breaded fish or smoked fish with deep fried potatoes and pickled vegetables.

Eating out will be made easier if the restaurant allows you the opportunity to make food choices that are migraine-friendly. You may need to make a special request that some food be prepared without seasonings to avoid additives. Choosing fresh fruit and vegetables from the list of allowed foods for migraine (see pp91–93) will help you avoid food that could trigger a migraine attack. Given below are suggestions for good food choices that will help you avoid a migraine attack, as well as meals to be avoided because they may encourage or trigger an attack.

PASTA DISHES

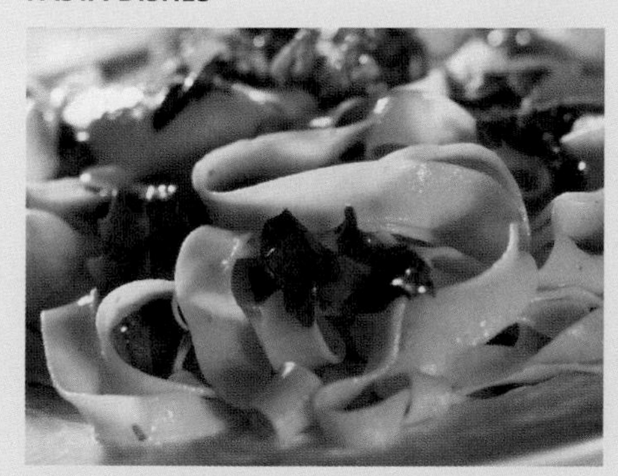

Good choices: Pasta with garlic and olive oil or butter, with grilled chicken or fish, accompanied by steamed vegetables or a spinach salad.

Bad choices: Sausage lasagne with matured cheese, salad with creamy Italian dressing and red wine. Spicy ramen noodles with barbequed pork.

SALAD DISHES

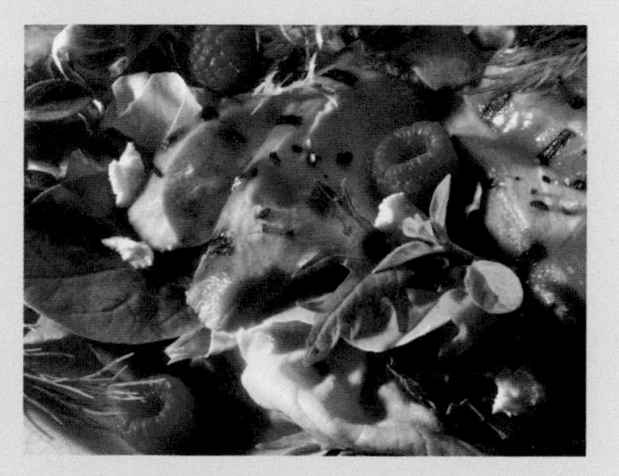

Good choices: Fresh spinach salad with grilled chicken, dried cranberries, fresh strawberries, and a raspberry vinaigrette dressing. Stuffed eggplant and garden salad with dressing. Fresh fruit for dessert.

Bad choices: Caesar salad, red wine, and chocolate dessert.

Migraine-friendly recipes

You can adapt many of your favorite recipes by replacing ingredients that are migraine triggers with more migraine-friendly ones. The more recipes you can adapt, the more dietary choices you will have. The following recipes come from a collection enjoyed by many of my migraine patients.

ITALIAN DRESSING

2 cups olive oil
1 cup vinegar
2 tbsp honey or sugar
1⅓ tbsp salt
1 tsp oregano
1 tsp basil
2 pinches cilantro
2 pinches black pepper
2 pinches minced garlic
1 pinch rosemary

Mix ingredients in blender. Refrigerate. If the dressing has congealed too much in the refrigerator, let it sit out for a few minutes, then shake or stir it to re-blend.

Yield: 3 cups

SALSA

2 cans tomatoes (32oz), drained (no MSG)
1 tsp onion flakes
1–3 tsp chopped garlic
1 can (4oz) diced green chilies
1 tbsp dried cilantro (optional)

Combine all ingredients in a blender. Process on "chop" for 15–30 seconds, depending on desired thickness.

Yield: about 2½ cups

TACO SEASONING MIX

1 tsp onion flakes
3 tsp chili powder
2 tsp salt
1 tsp flour
1 tsp dried red pepper
1 tsp garlic powder
1 tsp ground cumin
½ tsp oregano

Mix all ingredients together and store in airtight container.

Yield: ½ cup

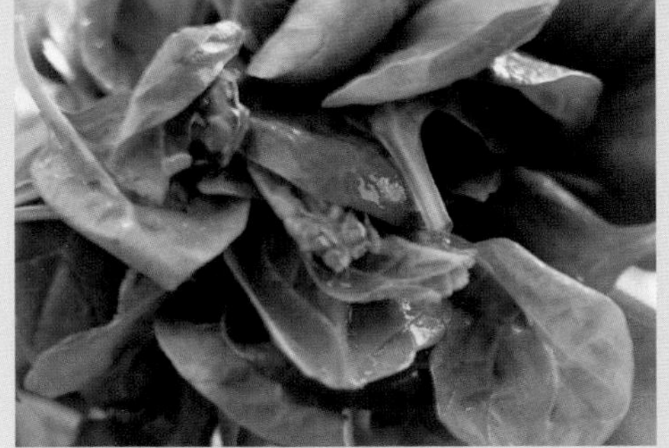

SWEETHEART SALAD

A bowl of fresh spinach

½ cup of dried cranberries

1 apple, diced small

2 cups chopped grilled chicken

¼ cup fresh mozzarella cheese

Toss all ingredients together in bowl and top with raspberry vinaigrette dressing.

Yield: 4 servings

TACO SALAD

½ lb ground beef or ground turkey

½ tsp chili powder

½ tsp garlic powder

½ tsp salt

½ head of lettuce, chopped

3 tomatoes, chopped

4oz grated American cheese

3oz tortilla chips

¾ cup salsa (see recipe, p168)

Cook meat with the seasonings in a greased skillet. Remove from heat. In a large bowl mix the lettuce, onion, tomatoes, cheese, and meat. Divide tortilla chips on 5 individual plates. Top with salad, then salsa.

Yield: 10 cups plus tortilla chips

VEGETABLE PITA SANDWICH

1 small zucchini, sliced

1 red pepper, sliced

1 tsp onion flakes

¼ tsp dried parsley

⅛ tsp dried thyme

⅛ tsp salt

Dash of pepper

2 wholewheat pita breads

½ cup cream cheese

In a greased skillet stir-fry vegetables and seasonings until vegetables are cooked to your liking. Cut pita bread in half and microwave on high for 20 seconds or until warm. Place 2 tbsp cream cheese into each pita. Fill with stir-fried vegetables.

Yield: 4 half sandwiches

PROTEIN PANCAKES

3 eggs

¼ tsp salt

¼ tsp vanilla

¼ cup rice protein powder

1 cup cottage cheese

¼ cup milk

1 cup flour

2 tbsp sugar

Combine first 6 ingredients in blender. Blend until smooth. Add flour and sugar and blend until smooth. On a greased griddle, cook pancakes until golden on both sides.

Yield: 12 pancakes (4-inch each)

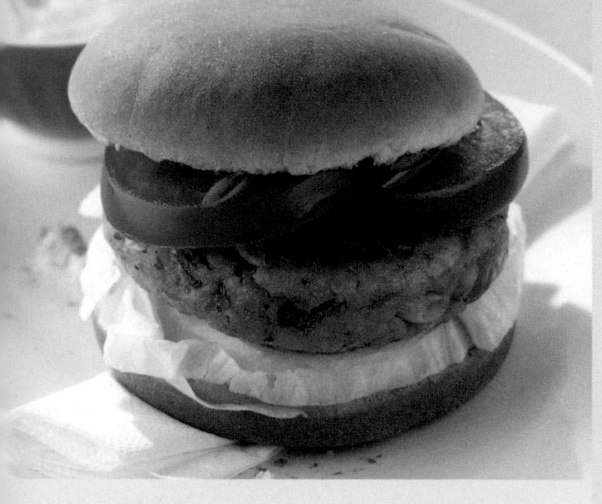

TUNA BURGERS

6oz of water-canned tuna, drained

2 tbsp mayonnaise

1 tsp dried parsley

½ tsp onion powder

2 drops Tabasco sauce

3 saltines

2 hamburger buns

Flake tuna and mix with remaining ingredients, except buns. Form into 2 patties and proceed with one of the methods below.

Conventional Oven: Preheat oven to 350°F. Arrange patties on a greased baking sheet. Bake for 25 minutes or until golden brown.

Stove Top: On a greased griddle or large skillet, cook each patty a few minutes on each side until golden brown.

Heat buns in oven or microwave until warm. Serve patties on hamburger buns.

Yield: 2 servings

OVEN-BAKED FISH

2lb fish fillets (sole, cod, or haddock)

¼ cup canola oil

1 tsp onion flakes

5 medium potatoes (cut into 1in pieces)

½ tsp salt

½ tsp pepper

1 tsp oregano

½ can (14 oz) tomatoes

14 fl oz water

Preheat oven to 350°F. Place potatoes on a greased pan; sprinkle with onion flakes, salt, pepper, and oregano. Roast for 10 minutes. Add tomatoes and water. Cover and bake until potatoes are almost done, about 45 minutes. Place fish on top. Bake for 20 minutes without cover.

Yield: 6 servings

PITA PIZZA

1 pita

2 tbsp tomato paste

¼ red pepper (diced)

¼ cup fresh mozzarella

1 chicken breast (cooked and diced)

¼ tsp oregano

Spread tomato paste on the pita, then place the diced red peppers and diced chicken on top. Sprinkle with the cheese and top off with oregano. Bake at 425°F in the oven for 8–10 minutes.

Yield: 1 serving

CHICKEN AND PEPPERS

1lb boneless, skinless chicken breasts
1 tsp cumin
¾ cup salsa (see recipe, p168)
½ tsp chopped garlic
1 tsp onion flakes
1 green pepper, sliced

Cut the chicken into 1-inch strips; sprinkle with cumin. Grease skillet with canola or olive oil and stir fry chicken strips until tender and no longer pink. Add salsa (see recipe), onion flakes, and green peppers. Cover and simmer for 10 minutes or until vegetables are tender.

Yield: 4 servings

CHICKEN CASSEROLE

4 chicken breasts with bone (boiled, pulled off bone, and shredded)
1 bag broccoli florets (cooked)
1 cup canola mayonnaise
Cream soup mix (see recipe below)
½ cup shredded American cheese
3 tbsp dried breadcrumbs

Cream Soup Mix:

½ cup dried milk (no soy product or MSG)
3 tbsp flour
1½ tbsp onion flakes
Dash of pepper
½ tsp dried basil
½ tsp dried thyme
1 tbsp chicken broth (no MSG)

Combine all ingredients in a saucepan and mix well. Add 2½ cups of cold water and stir over low heat until thickened. Let it cool. Combine with the canola mayonnaise. Preheat oven to 350°F. Take a 9×12 inch casserole dish and layer broccoli, chicken, soup mix, and American cheese; top with breadcrumbs. Bake for 30 minutes.

Yield: 4–6 servings

CARROT CAKE

2 cups plain flour
2 cups sugar
2 tsp baking soda
2 tsp cinnamon
4 eggs
1¼ cups of cooking oil
3 cups grated carrots

Icing:

1 stick butter (4oz)
8oz cream cheese (softened)
1 box powdered sugar (16oz)
1 tsp vanilla

Sift together the flour, sugar, baking soda, and cinnamon. Add eggs and oil and fold in the grated carrots. Pour mixture into three 8-inch round pans greased and sprinkled with flour. Bake at 350°F for 35 minutes.

To make the icing, mix cheese and butter with vanilla. Stir in the sugar. Allow the cake layers to cool, then spread the icing on top of each layer and stack the layers.

Women's health

Q I have severe menstrual migraine. What I can do to reduce the likelihood of having attacks?

It may be helpful to track menstrual cycles on your migraine diary. The falling estrogen levels, which occur 2–3 days before the first day of menstruation, trigger the menstrual migraine. You need to start your menstrual migraine treatment before the onset of the attack.

Q Even if I am unable to avoid a menstrual migraine, is there anything I can do to decrease the severity?

By avoiding migraine triggers, maintaining your exercise and relaxation routine, and reducing some of your activities, you can reduce the severity of your menstrual migraine and make it easier to abort. If you know that you are premenstrual by tracking your cycles, then you will be better able to make the changes.

Q Can I take my abortive therapy before the attack?

Using abortive therapy, specifically NSAIDs and triptans, daily for 3–4 days before the menstrual attack can be very helpful. You need to discuss this approach with the doctor who is treating you. The avoidance of migraine triggers during the week before menstruation is very important. By avoiding triggers and using the abortive medications you may be able to avoid the attack.

Q I have friends who take continuous oral contraceptives to prevent a menstrual migraine. Is that something I could do as well?

The use of oral contraceptives to treat menstrual migraine can be very helpful. Taking these contraceptives without a break means that estrogen levels in the blood do not fall or that the drop is less rapid. Since menstrual migraine is caused by the falling estrogen level, continuous use of contraceptives prevents the attack. You will need to discuss the use of continuous oral contraceptives with your gynecologist to know if it is a treatment option for you.

Q Sometimes I don't have menstrual migraine, but I do feel anxious and depressed during menstruation. Is this migraine or PMS?

That is a very good question, one I am not sure your gynecologist or a neurologist could answer. There is significant overlap between premenstrual migraine and premenstrual syndrome. They may be separate serotonin conditions or symptoms of the same serotonin–estrogen related condition. Many women experience both, and the treatment options are nearly identical.

Q How can I help my friends and family to better understand my menstrual migraine?

You can provide them with information regarding menstrual migraine and how changes in estrogen levels trigger a migraine attack. Family and friends, especially women, may be very interested in learning about estrogen and how it affects brain function. Some of your friends may simply need the reassurance that you are doing everything you can to feel well.

Q "Not tonight honey, I have a headache." Is having a headache a legitimate reason for not having sex?

It depends upon the severity of the migraine attack. A mild migraine attack could be aborted by the endorphins that are released during intercourse. A more severe attack with nausea and vomiting would make it difficult to do anything, let alone have sex. Coital headache is a type of headache that can occur during sexual climax. It can be easily treated by taking indometacin an hour before sexual intercourse.

Q If I have migraine can I use oral contraceptives?

Oral contraceptives containing estrogen can make women who have migraine with aura more vulnerable to stroke, so it depends on the number of other risk factors you have. Risk factors include: age over 45 years, smoking, hypertension, heart disease, and diabetes. If you have migraine without aura and no other risk factors, then a low-dose estrogen oral contraceptive can be taken.

Dealing with illnesses

Q What should I do if I have a headache that is not like my usual migraine headaches?

Any headache that starts very rapidly and is very severe needs immediate medical attention to make sure you have not had a brain hemorrhage (bleeding into the brain) from an aneurysm (abnormal ballooning of an artery wall) or stroke. A headache associated with fever and stiff neck also needs immediate attention as it can be caused by meningitis. When in doubt about a change in your usual headache patterns, it is important that you see a doctor.

Q How does having a chronic illness such as high blood pressure, asthma, or diabetes affect my migraine treatment?

If you have any other chronic illnesses apart from migraine, make sure that all your doctors are aware of your migraine. Your migraine medications must be safe to use with your chronic illnesses. In addition, review the medications for your chronic illness with the doctor treating your migraine to make sure that none could trigger an attack. Your exercise and relaxation program will benefit all your chronic illnesses. Your migraine diet may be a challenge if it has to be combined with the dietary restrictions of another illness, but you can get help from a nutritionist in working out different dietary requirements.

Q How do I prevent a migraine when I have a cold, flu, or other acute illness?

The most important thing you can do to avoid a migraine attack when you have an acute illness is to have plenty of fluids. When you are ill, dehydration and hypoglycemia are especially likely to trigger an attack. If your illness causes nausea, you must stop the vomiting so that you can continue your migraine medications, eat, and drink. Before you take medication for an acute illness, you must make sure it will not complicate your migraine care.

Q What will I need to do for my migraine if I have a surgical or dental procedure?

When you undergo a surgical procedure in which a general anesthetic will be used, you will be asked to fast for 12 hours before the procedure. The combination of fasting before the procedure and the post-procedure pain, along with the use of painkillers, may cause a migraine attack. During dental or minor surgical procedures, if epinephrine is added to the local anesthetic, an attack is likely. Ask your dentist or doctor if it is possible to avoid epinephrine. It is important that you resume eating as soon as possible after the operation and drink plenty of fluids. Analgesics often trigger migraine attacks, so try to avoid them after 48 hours. Ask your treating physician if you can use NSAIDs for your post-procedure pain.

Q I have suffered from depression and migraine for years. Are these conditions related?

Yes, there is a connection between depression and migraine, but they do not lead to one another. The connection is thought to be genetic. Both illnesses can be inherited, and both are caused by a disturbance in the levels of serotonin. There are several serotonin-related illnesses—you will probably recognize many of these conditions, either because you have them or because someone else in your family does. These illnesses include, but are not limited to, anxiety, depression, insomnia, attention deficit disorder, irritable bowel syndrome, fibromyalgia, and restless legs syndrome.

Q Is it necessary for me to search out specific treatment for each of my serotonin-related illnesses?

Yes, you need to see the appropriate expert for treatment of your individual serotonin-related illnesses. Although the conditions are caused by a disturbance in serotonin, the medications used to treat each illness can be very different. Your migraine-friendly lifestyle can help because stress management and exercise increase serotonin levels.

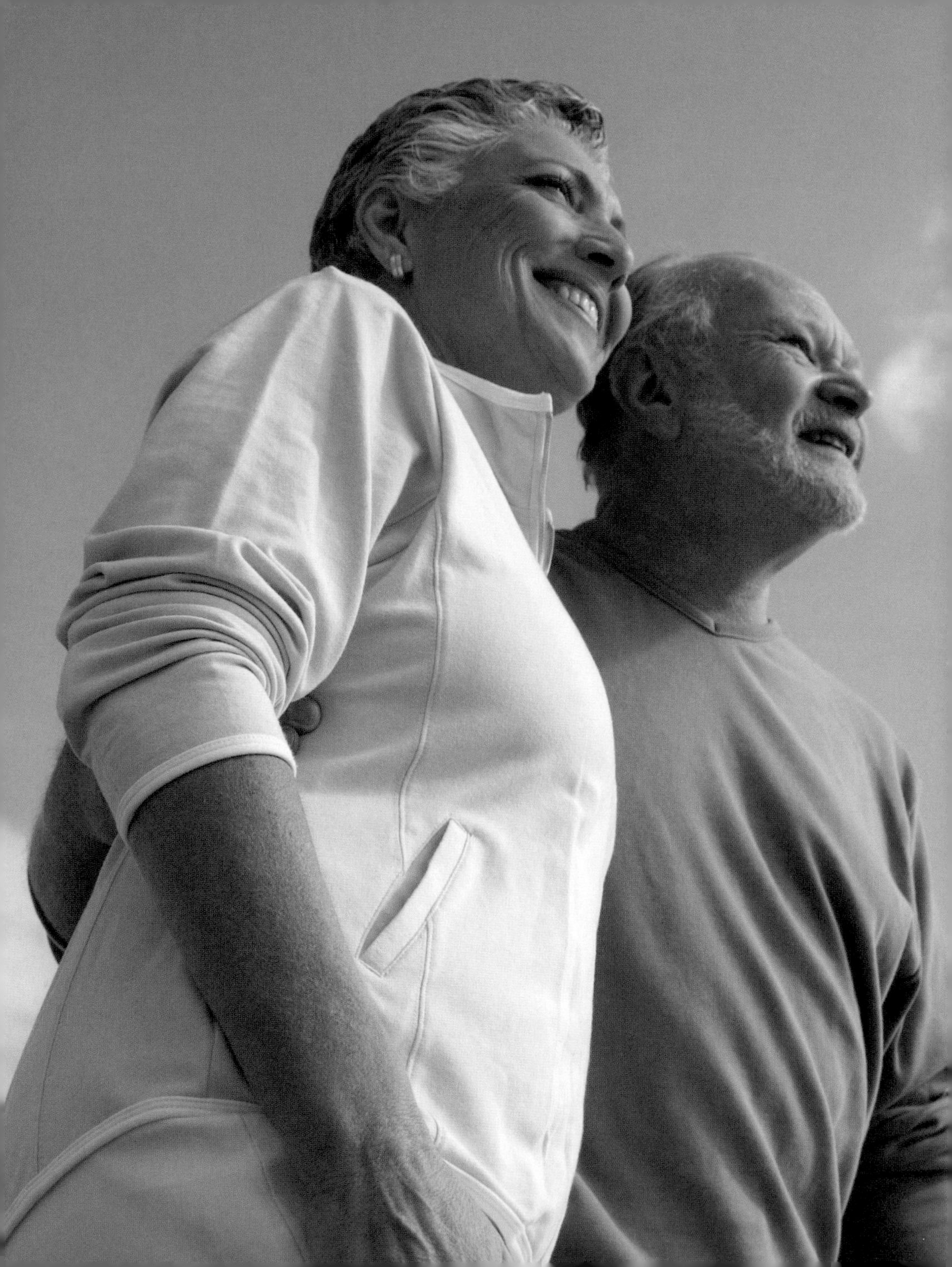

Long-term outlook

No one can predict the future. More importantly, no one can promise you a cure. However, recent discoveries in migraine research have provided us with more options than ever before for treating migraine effectively. The future for the migraine sufferer is very promising.

Long-term effects of migraine

Q Are there long-term physical side effects of migraine? Could it possibly lead to brain damage?

There is no evidence to suggest that having migraine causes any damage to the brain. There may be a very small increased risk of stroke for people who have migraine with aura (see p25). The exact reason for this increased risk is unknown, but it may be related to a congenital heart defect called patent foramen ovale. The risk of stroke does increase if a woman with migraine with aura is a smoker or is taking combined hormonal contraceptives.

Q Are there long-term psychological and social effects of migraine?

Left untreated, migraine causes significant suffering and disability. Poorly controlled migraine is associated with higher levels of unemployment and an increased risk of depression. Although our understanding of migraine has improved in recent years, little is known about the extent to which this chronic illness affects people's lives.

Q Will my migraine get worse if it isn't treated?

Yes, a progression of the condition is a very possible long-term effect of untreated migraine. For many years doctors involved in the treatment of headache patients have observed how some individuals experience more migraine attacks over time. As the attacks become more frequent they become more severe and last longer. For those who are given analgesics, their frequent migraine attacks quickly turn into chronic daily headache due to medication overuse.

Q I have developed chronic daily headache. What are my prospects for improvement?

With appropriate treatment, your headaches should decrease and you will revert back to intermittent migraine attacks that can be controlled with abortive therapy. I call this "neuroverting." As cardiac patients with heart rhythm problems are cardioverted with medication or by shocking the heart, headache patients can be "neuroverted" out of a chronic daily headache pattern with migraine treatment.

Q How can I prevent progression of my migraine?

You can prevent progression of your migraine by preventing migraine attacks. The longer you have migraine, the more likely it is to progress. It is important that your preventive therapy is effective. You need to reduce headache days to 2 a month or less; if you haven't achieved this you need to try another preventive medication or a combination of preventive medications.

Q Are there risk factors for disease progression in migraine?

Studies have shown that risk factors for migraine progression include: obesity, medication overuse headaches, and post-traumatic headaches. Aggressive treatment of these conditions will lessen the risk by decreasing the number of headaches. I believe excessive intake of carbohydrates triggers frequent migraine attacks that subsequently causes chronic migraine. Obesity and chronic migraine have a common link: excessive carbohydrates. If you decrease your carbohydrate intake you may notice a decrease in the frequency of your migraine attacks before weight loss.

Q What do I do if my current medical treatment is not working?

If you are having trouble controlling your attacks, you may need to see a specialist. There are many headache treatment centers in the US. You can find out more by visiting some of the websites listed on p184.

Long-term effects of medication

Q Are there any long-term effects from taking the medications used to treat migraine?

No long-term effects have been reported on the use of triptans. This class of drugs, used in abortive therapy, has been on the market in Europe since 1990 and on the US market since 1992. The nonsteroidal anti-inflammatory drugs (NSAIDs) may cause stomach ulcers, gastrointestinal bleeding, and kidney disease if used in excess for long periods. Analgesics can cause medication overuse headache and drug addiction if used daily.

Q Does this mean it is OK to take triptans every day?

Not exactly. Triptans or other abortive medications (such as NSAIDs) shouldn't be used daily. Although triptans do not seem to cause long-term effects, the overuse of any abortive medications could cause medication overuse headache (see pp78–81). In addition, overuse can make medications less effective. Abortive therapy is a very important part of migraine treatment but it cannot be your only treatment. You must also have a preventive treatment program in place. If you are using abortive therapy more than 2 days a week then preventive medication is needed.

Q How many times in a day can I use abortive therapy?

Since abortive therapy needs to be effective it shouldn't be required more than twice a day. You should ideally need it no more than once within a 24-hour period. If your migraine attack isn't aborted within 2 hours or less and you experience relapses within the following 24 hours, then you need to change your treatment.

Q I have been using analgesics for years for my daily headaches. How can I find help?

If you have used analgesics regularly for years, you will have developed medication overuse headache, which causes chronic daily headache. These conditions can be treated, but this is not easily done. You will need the expertise of a headache clinic and will need to make your treatment a priority in the same way as, say, a cancer patient does. You must become a headache survivor.

Q Are there any long-term effects from taking medications for migraine prevention?

Most medications used to prevent migraine have been on the market for years. The newest preventive medication, topirimate, has been on the market since 1997. Although every drug used to prevent migraine can have side effects, there have been no reported long-term effects yet.

Q I do not want to take medications long-term. Will there come a time when I do not need preventive medications?

When you have been able to decrease the frequency of your migraine attacks to less than twice a month for more than 8 months, you can try to slowly do away with preventive medications. You will need to work hard to maintain your dietary restrictions, follow your exercise and relaxation programs, and reduce stress if you are going to be successful at stopping your preventive medication.

Q What is the best way to stop my preventive medications?

When you and your doctor have made a decision that your migraine is controlled enough to stop preventive medications, you need to stop the medications very slowly. If you are taking several medications, you should stop one at a time. As you decrease the dose of your daily medication every 3–4 weeks, you need to track your migraine frequency very closely. If the attacks begin to increase in frequency, you must increase the dose of your medication by a small amount. Regain migraine control for at least 4 months before you try again to lower the dose.

The future of migraine

Q What does the future hold for migraine sufferers?

Migraine remains underdiagnosed in the US, where just half of some 28 million people with migraine have been properly diagnosed. Failure to recognize migraine and its misdiagnosis as another headache type are the most common reasons for this. Many migraine sufferers have been diagnosed with tension or sinus headache because their symptoms do not fit the regular criteria. Studies show that pain on both sides of the head, nonthrobbing pain, and pain at the back of the head and neck are common in migraine, but as these are generally associated with tension (stress) headaches, this diagnosis may be made instead. The medical community and the public need to be better educated about migraine and migraine sufferers.

Q Why are men generally not diagnosed as having migraine?

Studies have shown men are associated with a lower probability of being diagnosed with migraine. Men are reluctant to seek healthcare for any medical problem, and headaches are often assumed to be caused by stress.

Q What are the economic costs of migraine?

Migraine is a chronic illness that results in significant suffering and economic loss. It has been estimated that migraine affects nearly 6.2 million workers employed outside the home and results in lost productivity valued at 1.4 billion dollars per year. Studies show workdays lost annually to migraine ranging from 1.4 to 4, but none of the studies consider the impaired productivity of individuals who continue to work with a migraine attack. Experts estimate the annual indirect cost of migraine in the US to be between 1.4 and 17.2 billion dollars.

Q Will we ever have a fail-safe test for migraine?

I am sure that someday we will have a diagnostic test for migraine. Researchers have tried to find a biological marker on DNA but have found little, so far, that seems promising. The development of imaging studies may provide the first breakthrough. At present, the diagnosis is made by asking the headache sufferer about his or her history of headaches and the family history.

Q What are the recent advances in migraine?

Recent advances in the study of disease mechanisms and diagnosis have given us a better understanding of what causes migraine, and we are better able to choose the right medications to treat migraine attacks, rather than just treating the pain of a headache. The current theory of the multimechanism of migraine allows us to target different areas of the brain causing the attack. The combination of triptan and nonsteroidal anti-inflammatory drugs (NSAIDs) enables people to stop attacks more effectively.

Q Are there new treatments for migraine prevention?

Researchers are now turning their attention to migraine prevention. For years, medications developed to treat other diseases have been used to treat migraine. As we discover how the illness of migraine progresses and what may make certain individuals more vulnerable to its progression, we will be able to find improved treatment options. The future does hold much hope for the migraine sufferer.

Q What is the ultimate goal for migraine treatment?

Now that we understand migraine to be a progressive disease, achieving a pain-free outcome is the ultimate treatment goal of patients. A migraine attack must be treated early and aggressively to achieve the pain-free outcome within 2 hours. The longer an attack lasts, the more vulnerable you are to another attack.

Useful addresses

National Headache Foundation
(Includes physician finder)
820 N. Orleans, Suite 217
Chicago, IL 60610
Tel: (888) NHF-5552
Website: www.headaches.org

American Council for Headache Education
(Includes physician finder)
19 Mantua Road
Mt. Royal, NJ 08061
Tel: (856) 423-0258
Website: www.achenet.org

American Headache Society
19 Mantua Road
Mt. Royal, NJ 08061
Tel: (856) 423-0258
Website: www.americanheadachesociety.org

The National Migraine Association (MAGNUM)
113 South St. Asaph, Suite 100
Alexandria, VA 22314
Tel: (703) 349-1929
Website: www.migraines.org

Organization for Understanding Cluster Headaches (OUCH)
3225 Winding Way
Round Rock, TX 78664
Website: www.ouch-us.org

National Institute of Neurological Disorders and Stroke
NIH Neurological Institute
P. O. Box 5801
Bethesda, MD 20824
Tel: (800) 352-9424
TTY (for people using adaptive equipment): (301) 468-5981
Website: www.ninds.nih.gov

American Academy of Neurology
Website: www.thebrainmatters.org

American Academy of Family Physicians
Website: www.familydoctor.org

To find our more about the author, Carol A. Foster, MD:
Website: www.gottaheadache.com

Index

About the Author

Carol A. Foster, MD is a board-certified neurologist specializing in migraine and founder of the Valley Neurological Headache and Research Center in Phoenix, Arizona. A migraine sufferer herself, Dr. Foster completed her neurology residency at the Barrow Neurological Institute, St. Joseph's Hospital. She has since established her practice as a leading private clinic for the treatment of headache disorders. Dr. Foster is a regular reviewer for medical journals *Headache* and *Headache Quarterly* and author of several publications on headache. She has given a number of lectures and seminars on the topic of migraine.

Author's acknowledgments

I am so grateful to those at DK and to my editors, Philip Morgan and Andrea Bagg, who gave me this opportunity. To the headache sufferers, who have taught me most of the information contained in these pages. And for those who love and support me, my children Jennifer and Melissa, my family, my friends, and my office staff—your encouragement has meant everything. Most importantly, I thank God who helped me live it and then put it into words.

For the publishers

Dorling Kindersley would like to thank Jill Hamilton and Isabel de Cordova; also Fran Vargo for picture research.

Picture credits

The publisher would like to thank the following for their kind permission to reproduce their photographs: (Key: a-above; b-below/bottom; c-centre; l-left; r-right; t-top)

2 Getty Images: Riser/Thomas Northcut. **7** Corbis: Andrew Brookes (r). Getty Images: Taxi/Diane Padys (c). Masterfile: Noel Hendrickson (l). **8** Getty Images: altrendo images. **12** Getty Images: The Image Bank/Sacha Ajbeszyc. **16** Delia Malchert: (l) (r). **17** Getty Images: Photonica/Mark Adams. **18** Getty Images: Photonica/Emmet Malmstrom (l). Masterfile: Noel Hendrickson (r). **19** Alamy Images: Bubbles Photolibrary. **28** Getty Images: Stone/Ryan MacVay. **36** Corbis: zefa/A. Inden. **42** Corbis: LWA-Dann Tardif. **46** Science Photo Library: AJ Photo. **52** Corbis: Jose Luis Pelaez, Inc. **55** Corbis: zefa/Larry Williams. **62** Getty Images: Stone/Bruce Ayres. **68** Masterfile: Chad Johnston. **72** Getty Images: Photographer's Choice/Kevin Summers (l); StockFood Creative/Dick Frank (r). **73** Getty Images: The Image Bank/Anthony Johnson (b); StockFood Creative/Werner Blessing (t). **80** Photolibrary: Phototake Inc. **82** Getty Images: Stone/Peter Correz. **87** Corbis: Jerry Tobias. **93** Getty Images: StockFood Creative/Roger Stowell (c). **100** Getty Images: Iconica/Fat Chance Productions. **102** Corbis: zefa/Mika. **104** Corbis: Michael Keller. **112** Corbis: Norbert Schaefer. **113** Getty Images: The Image Bank/Darren Robb. **121** Corbis: Andrew Brookes. **124** Getty Images: Stone/Ian O'Leary. **127** Corbis: Chuck Savage. **131** Corbis: Michael Keller. **132** Science Photo Library: AJ Photo. **133** Corbis: Tom Stewart (c); zefa/G. Baden (b). **142** Getty Images: Riser/Bruce Ayres. **148** Getty Images: Stone/Donna Day. **160** Getty Images: Riser/Larry Dale Gordon. **162** Getty Images: Robert Harding World Imagery. **163** Getty Images: Stone/Robert Warren. **166** Corbis: photocuisine/P.Desgrieux (l). Getty Images: StockFood Creative/Elizabeth Watt (r). **167** Getty Images: Taxi/Prima Press (l); Taxi/Diane Padys (r). **168** Corbis: photocuisine/J.Bilic. **169** Getty Images: StockFood Creative/Roger Stowell. **170** Getty Images: StockFood Creative/Klaus Arras. **176** Corbis: zefa/Fabio Cardoso